Understanding Medical Terms

A self-instructional course

Ralph Rickards, M.A., D.Phil.
Marketing Director
Cambridge Communication Limited

Churchill Livingstone
EDINBURGH LONDON & NEW YORK 1980

CHURCHILL LIVINGSTONE
Medical Division of the Longman Group Limited

Distributed in the United States of America by
Churchill Livingstone Inc., 1560 Broadway, New York,
N.Y. 10036, and by associated companies, branches and
representatives throughout the world.

First published 1980
  Reprinted 1986

ISBN 0-443-02029-9

British Library Cataloguing in Publication Data

Rickards, Ralph
    Understanding medical terms
    1. Medicine—Terminology—Programmed
instruction
    I. Title
    610'.1'4   R123   80-40489

Produced by Longman Singapore Publishers Pte Ltd.
Printed in Singapore

About this book

Something like three-quarters of the terms used in medicine and its associated disciplines are of Greek or Latin origin. These languages are no longer widely studied. Consequently many newcomers to medical and paramedical subjects find that they have to cope with a whole new vocabulary, as well as learn the unfamiliar concepts of their subject.

This book attempts to overcome this problem by providing a simple guide to the origin and formation of medical terms. It should help the learner to acquire a basic vocabulary and should make it easier to understand new terms when he or she meets with them. The book should be useful to medical students, nurses, laboratory workers, medical secretaries, medical representatives and others whose work or interests involve using and understanding medical terms.

The book is not a medical text book and does not claim to provide a short cut to the mastery of medicine or any related subjects. The book is not exhaustive but has been kept short, simple and useful by including only more commonly used terms. Finally the book has been designed for the learner of medical terms and not for authorities on language; it may therefore not be totally linguistically accurate.

How to use this book

The book is divided into a number of short sections, each of which is followed by a test. To use the book you simply read through a section and then do the test. The test questions are usually based on information given in the previous section, but they may require you to recall information supplied earlier in the book, or to apply your general knowledge.

When you have answered all the questions for a section you should check your answers. If your answers are all correct continue working through the book. If any of your answers are wrong read the appropriate information and the question again and make sure that you understand the correct answer before continuing to work through the book.

Part one - Introduction

Anyone who comes across complex medical terms for the first time is likely
to be utterly perplexed. Words like otorhinolaryngology, electroencephalography,
and pseudohypoparathyroidism appear to defy pronunciation let alone
comprehension! However, complex terms like these are built up from simpler,
smaller parts. If the meanings of the smaller parts are known, it is often possible
to deduce the sense of a complex term.

For example, the word otorhinolaryngology can be broken down as follows:

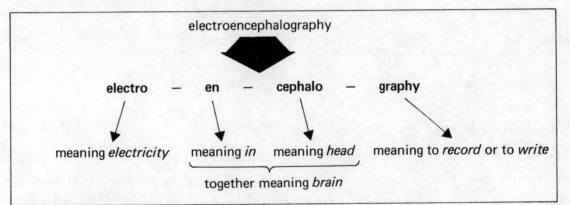

Therefore **otorhinolaryngology** means the study of the ears, nose and larynx.

The other two words above can be analysed in a similar way:

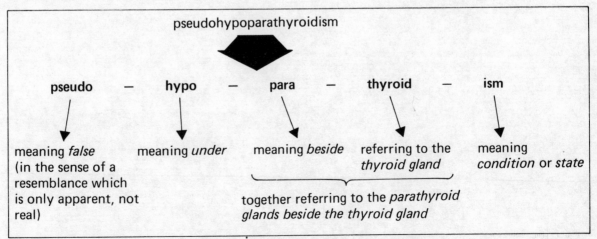

Therefore **electroencephalography** means the recording of the electrical activity
of the brain.

Therefore **pseudohypoparathyroidism** means a condition resembling underactivity
of the parathyroid glands.

The parts from which the words of the medical vocabulary are constructed are of three types. The *root* forms the basis of a word, Other parts are added to the root to modify its meaning. *Prefixes* are syllables added in front of a root to modify it. *Suffixes* are syllables added after a root to modify it.

Roots, prefixes and suffixes are usually of Greek or Latin origin.

Strictly speaking, Greek roots should have only Greek prefixes and suffixes, and Latin roots should have only Latin prefixes and suffixes. However, there are some exceptions which have crept into the vocabulary, to the anger of some linguists.

In order to have the foundations for understanding a large number of medical terms it is only necessary to know the meanings of comparatively few roots, prefixes and suffixes. This is because the number of these terms in common use is quite small, although the number of different ways in which they can be combined is enormous.

TEST

1. From what you have read so far deduce the meanings of the following medical terms:

   (a) encephalology

   (b) hypolarynx

   (c) otography.

2. Which of the statements on the right apply to the terms listed on the left?

   (a) Root   (i) Modifies the meaning of the basis of a word

   (b) Prefix   (ii) Comes at the end of a word

   (c) Suffix   (iii) Forms the basis of a word

                    (iv) Comes at the beginning of a word

3. Describe briefly the process by which the meaning of a complex medical term can be deduced from a knowledge of the meanings of the roots, prefixes and suffixes.

6

ANSWERS TO TEST

1. (a) Encephalology is the study of the brain (including its functions and diseases).

    (b) The hypolarynx is the underpart of the larynx.

    (c) Otography means a description of (writing about) the ear.

2. (a) (iii)

    (b) (i) (iv)

    (c) (i) (ii)

3. (i) The complex medical term is split up into its component prefix(es), root(s) and suffix(es).

    (ii) The meaning of each of the components is established.

    (iii) The meanings of the components are put together to give the meaning of the complete term.

BIOLOGY AND ITS BRANCHES

The principles of word construction and analysis outlined on the previous pages can be illustrated by looking at some of the terms used for different branches of medical science.

The study of living things forms the subject of **biology** (from the Greek words **bios**, meaning *life*, and **logos**, meaning *science* or *study*). The root **bio-** appears in many related words:

biochemistry	—	the study of the chemical processes involved in life;
biophysics	—	the study of the physical processes involved in life;
micro**bio**logy	—	the study of micro-organisms (small life);
anti**bio**tic	—	a substance capable of destroying life (especially bacterial life).

An important branch of biology is the science of the functions of living things, or **physiology** (from the Greek words **physis**, meaning *nature,* and **logos**). The root **phys-** (or **phy-** or **physi-**) appears in words like:

physics	—	the science dealing with the properties of matter and energy;
physical	—	according to the laws of nature;
physician	—	one who practises medicine (presumably by applying the study of nature).

The branch of biology which deals with the structure of the body is known as **anatomy**. This word is derived from the Greek words **ana**, meaning *up* or *back,* and **tome**, meaning *cutting*. The derivation reveals that the study of anatomy is largely based on dissection, or cutting up.

Two subjects closely related to anatomy are **histology,** the study of the structure of the tissues of the body (from the Greek words **histos**, meaning *web* or *tissue,* and **logos**), and **cytology,** the study of cells (from the Greek words **cytos**, meaning *cell,* and **logos**).

TEST

4. Which of the definitions on the right apply to the terms listed on the left?

(a) Cytobiology   (i) Description of the tissues

(b) Microtomy   (ii) The study of the chemical processes in tissues

(c) Histochemistry   (iii) Cutting of thin sections

(d) Histography   (iv) The study of the chemical processes in cells

(e) Cytochemistry   (v) The study of the life of cells

5. Deduce the subject matter of the following scientific disciplines

(a) Biomathematics

(b) Cytophysics.

6. Complete the following sentence:

Erythro**cytes**, leuco**cytes** and lympho**cytes** are different kinds of_____

8

MEDICINE AND ITS BRANCHES I

The word **medicine** is derived directly from the Latin word **medicina** and means the art, or science, of restoring and preserving health.

Many of the specialities into which medicine is divided are named by the addition of the suffix **-logy** to the appropriate root. Examples include:

dermato**logy**	— the branch of medicine concerned with the skin (from the Greek **derma**, meaning *skin*);
gynaeco**logy**	— the branch of medicine concerned with women (from the Greek **gyne**, meaning *woman*);
patho**logy**	— the study of disease (especially the structural and functional changes in tissues caused by disease) (from the Greek **pathos** meaning *suffering*);
psycho**logy**	— the study of behaviour (from the Greek **psyche**, meaning *soul* or *spirit*).

Other branches of medicine are named by the addition of the suffixes **-iatry** or **-iatrics** to the appropriate root. These suffixes are derived from the Greek word **iatros**, meaning *physician*. Examples include:

ger**iatrics**	— the branch of medicine concerned with old people (from the Greek **geras**, meaning *old age*);
paed**iatrics**	— the branch of medicine concerned with children (from the Greek **pais**, meaning *child*);
psych**iatry**	— the treatment of mental disorders.

TEST

7.   Deduce the meanings of the following terms:
     (a)   Neurophysiology
     (b)   Neurology
     (c)   Neuropathy
           (The Greek word **neuron** means *nerve*).

8.   What would you expect to be the cause of an **iatrogenic** disorder?

9.   Which of the definitions on the right apply to the terms listed on the left?

     (a)   Gynecopathy   (i)   The treatment of mental disorders
     (b)   Psychiatry   (ii)   A disease peculiar to women
     (c)   Psychology   (iii) The study of old people
     (d)   Psychopathology   (iv)   The study of mental disorders
     (e)   Gerontology   (v)   The study of behaviour.

10

MEDICINE AND ITS BRANCHES II

The study of medicine often involves the study of the causes of disease, or
aetiology (from the Greek words **aetia**, meaning *cause*, and **logos**).

The practice of medicine employs the arts of **diagnosis** and **prognosis**. Both of
these words are derived from the Greek word **gnosis**, meaning *knowledge* or
judgement. The prefix **dia** means *through* or *about*, hence **diagnosis** means
knowledge about and is used in medicine in the sense of the identification of
a disease.

The prefix **pro** means *before*, hence **prognosis** means *foreknowledge* and is
used in medicine in the sense of forecasting the course of a disease. The word
pathognomonic has a similar root, **gnomon** meaning *indicator*. It is used to
refer to a sign or symptom which is characteristic of a particular disease.

The purpose of medicine is healing. The Greek for *to heal* is **therapeuein**,
from which the words **therapy** and **therapeutics** are derived. The suffix -**therapy**
meaning *treatment*, appears in many words, for example:

physio**therapy**	—	the treatment of disease by natural agencies (such as heat or sunlight);
hydro**therapy**	—	the treatment of disease by the application of water (from the Greek words **hydro** meaning *water*, and **therapeuein**);
chemo**therapy**	—	the treatment of disease by chemicals.

Although the strict meaning of the term **chemotherapy** is the treatment of disease by chemicals, the word is commonly used in the more restricted sense of the use of a chemical agent to kill an infective organism or cancerous cell. Chemotherapy is therefore a branch of **pharmacotherapy,** the treatment of disease by drugs. **Pharmacotherapy** is derived from the Greek word **pharmakon,** meaning *drug* (or *poison* or *spell*). This word appears as a root in such words as:

pharmaceutical	—	pertaining to drugs;
pharmacist	—	druggist;
pharmacology	—	the study of drugs;
pharmacopeia	—	a book containing details of products used in medicine (from the Greek words **pharmakon** and **poiein,** meaning *to make*).
pharmacy	—	the preparation and dispensing of drugs; or a druggist's shop.

Finally, there is one important branch of medicine which has not yet been mentioned, namely **surgery.** This word is derived from the Greek words **cheir,** meaning *hand,* and **ergon,** meaning *work,* by way of the early English word **chirurgery.**

TEST

10. Deduce the meanings of the following terms:

(a) Electrotherapy

(b) Radiotherapy

(c) Physiatrics

11. Define:

(a) Aetiology

(b) Pharmacology

(c) Neurosurgery.

12. What is the difference between the meanings of the words *diagnosis* and *prognosis?*

12

Part two - The body

INTRODUCTION

In this section annotated diagrams are used to show the roots from which medical terms referring to the body are constructed. In the annotations the commonly used English word is shown in capital letters. The appropriate roots derived from Greek and Latin are shown underneath the English word. Any relevant notes are added underneath the Greek and/or Latin roots.

Where more than two roots are in common use, all the roots are shown in the appropriate typeface. Where only one root is in common use, only that root is shown. For example:

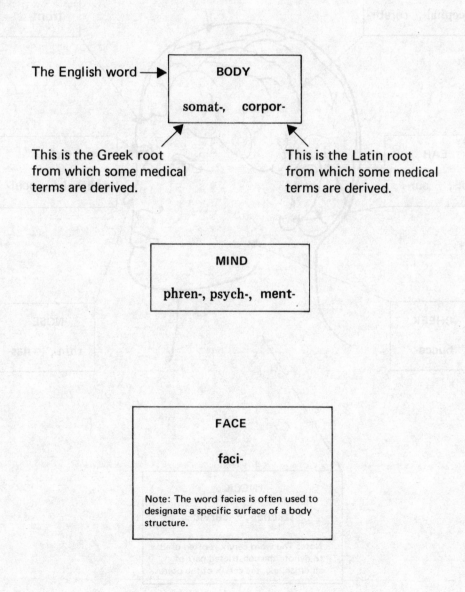

The English word → BODY

somat-,   corpor-

This is the Greek root from which some medical terms are derived.

This is the Latin root from which some medical terms are derived.

MIND

phren-, psych-, ment-

FACE

faci-

Note: The word facies is often used to designate a specific surface of a body structure.

14

THE HEAD

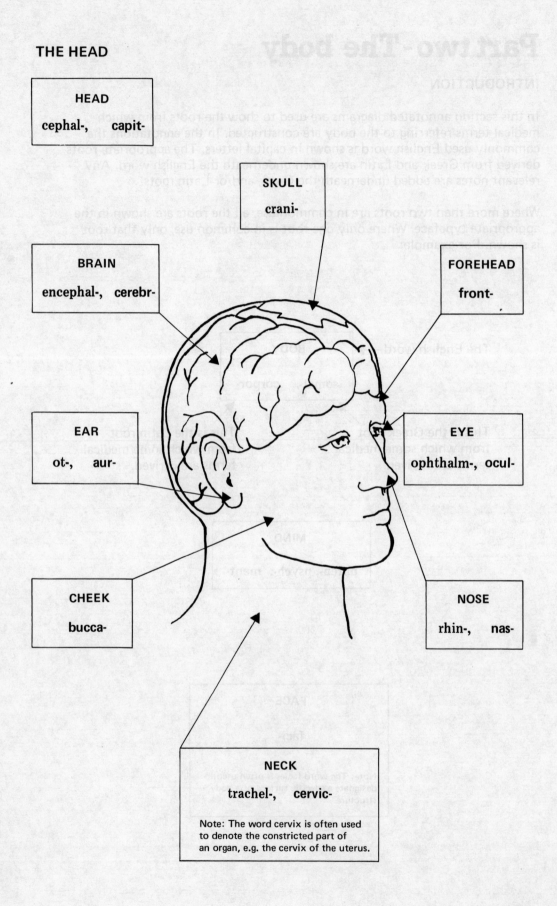

HEAD

cephal-, capit-

SKULL

crani-

BRAIN

encephal-, cerebr-

FOREHEAD

front-

EAR

ot-, aur-

EYE

ophthalm-, ocul-

CHEEK

bucca-

NOSE

rhin-, nas-

NECK

trachel-, cervic-

Note: The word cervix is often used
to denote the constricted part of
an organ, e.g. the cervix of the uterus.

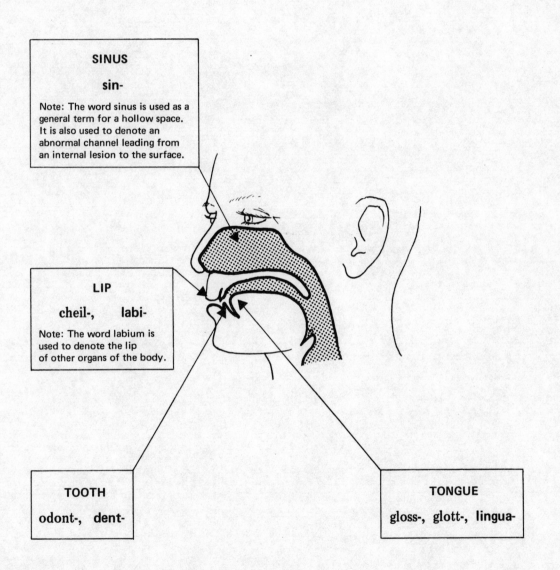

MOUTH

stom(at)-,   or-

Note: The word stoma is used to mean any mouth-like opening onto a surface.

SINUS

sin-

Note: The word sinus is used as a general term for a hollow space. It is also used to denote an abnormal channel leading from an internal lesion to the surface.

LIP

cheil-,   labi-

Note: The word labium is used to denote the lip of other organs of the body.

TOOTH

odont-, dent-

TONGUE

gloss-, glott-, lingua-

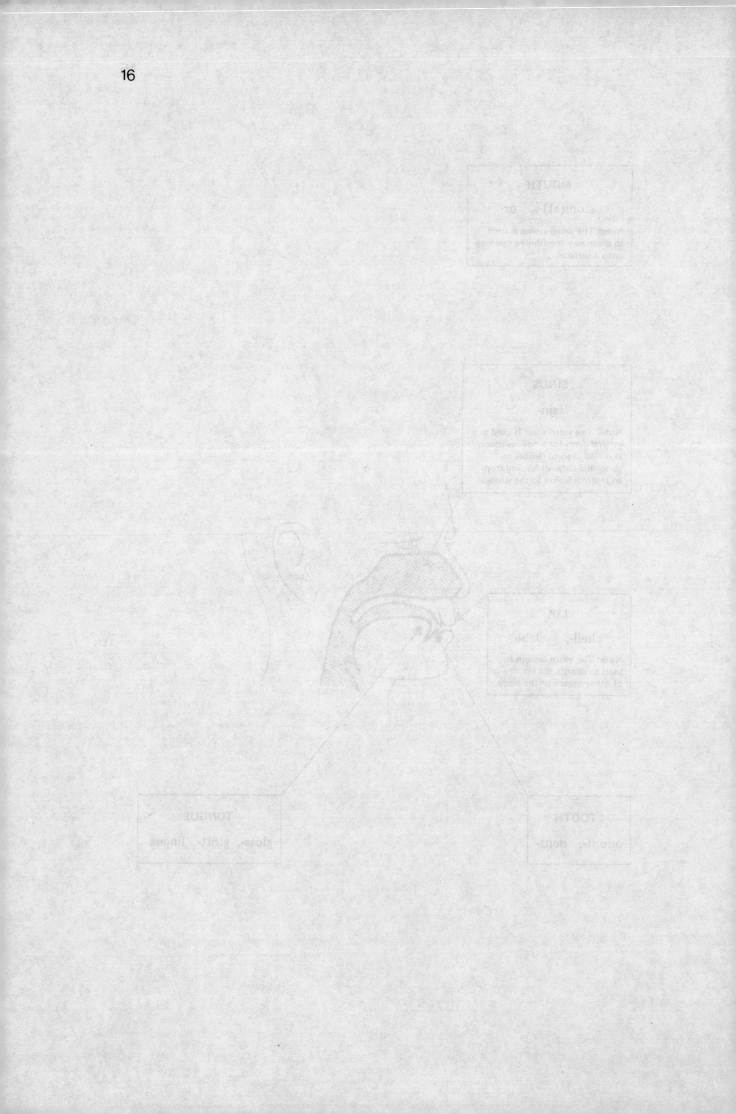

TEST

13. Which of the diseases on the right affect the parts of the body listed on the left?

(a) Nose   (i) Stomatitis
(b) Lip   (ii) Ophthalmia
(c) Ear   (iii) Perennial rhinitis
(d) Mouth   (iv) Otitis media
(e) Tongue   (v) Cheilocarcinoma
(f) Eye   (vi) Glossitis

14. Which parts of the body do the following nerves supply?

(a) Oculomotor nerve
(b) Lingual nerve
(c) Buccal nerve
(d) Labial nerve.

15. Deduce the meanings of the following adjectives:

(a) Somatic
(b) Phrenic
(c) Cephalic
(d) Cranial
(e) Dental
(f) Cervical
(g) Cerebral.

16. On which parts of the body are the following instruments used?

(a) Ophthalmoscope
(b) Auriscalpium
(c) Craniometer
(d) Odontoglyph
(e) Encaphalometer.

18

ANSWERS TO TEST

13.   (a)   (iii)
           (b)   (v)
           (c)   (iv)
           (d)   (i)
           (e)   (vi)
           (f)   (ii)

14.   (a)   The eye
           (b)   The tongue
           (c)   The cheek
           (d)   The lip

15.   (a)   Pertaining to the body
           (b)   Pertaining to the mind   (Phrenic can also mean pertaining to the diaphragm, a consequence of the Greek idea that the mind and diaphragm were related)
           (c)   Pertaining to the head
           (d)   Pertaining to the skull
           (e)   Pertaining to the teeth
           (f)   Pertaining to the neck   (or any cervix)
           (g)   Pertaining to the brain.

16.   (a)   The eye
           (b)   The ear
           (c)   The skull
           (d)   The teeth
           (e)   The brain

THE TRUNK AND LIMBS

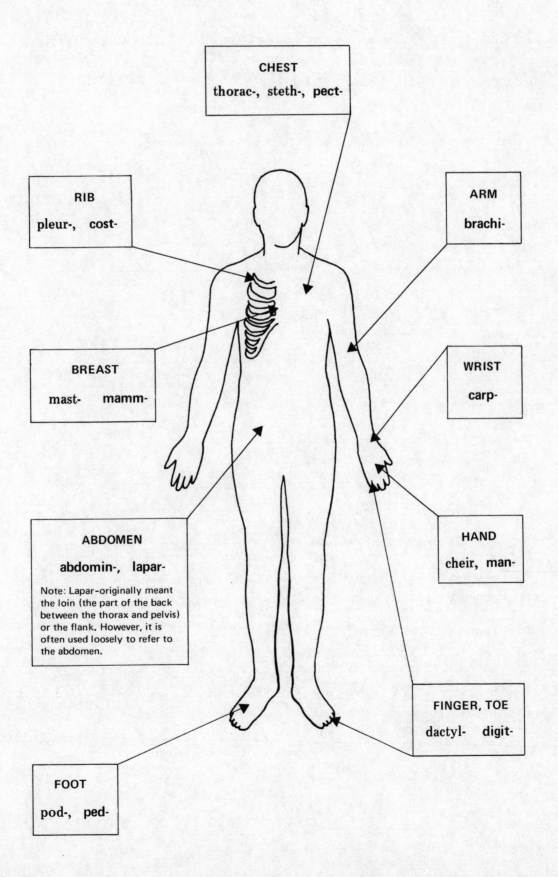

CHEST
thorac-, steth-, pect-

RIB
pleur-, cost-

ARM
brachi-

BREAST
mast- mamm-

WRIST
carp-

ABDOMEN

abdomin-, lapar-

Note: Lapar-originally meant
the loin (the part of the back
between the thorax and pelvis)
or the flank. However, it is
often used loosely to refer to
the abdomen.

HAND
cheir, man-

FINGER, TOE
dactyl- digit-

FOOT
pod-, ped-

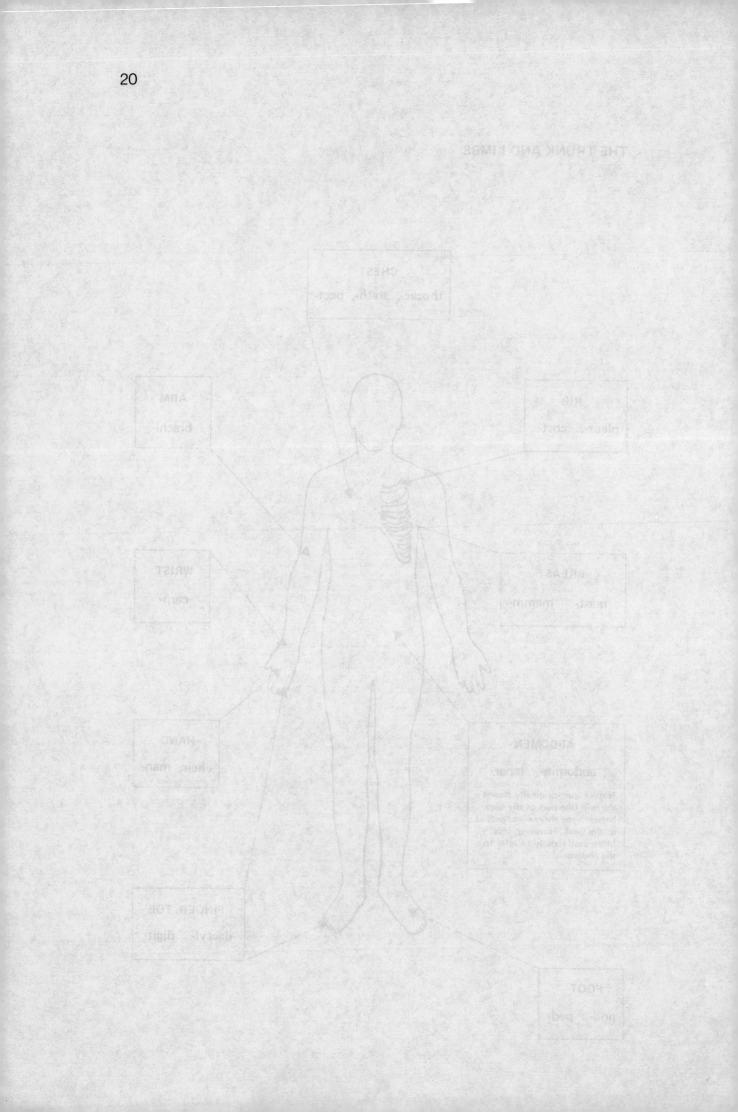

TEST

17. Whereabouts in the body are the following?

(a) Carpal bones

(b) Brachial artery

(c) Pectoral muscles

(d) Mammary glands

(e) Intercostal muscles.

18. On which parts of the body are the following surgical procedures carried out?

(a) Laparotomy

(b) Mastectomy

(c) Thoracocentesis

(d) Cheiroplasty.

22

THE CARDIOVASCULAR SYSTEM

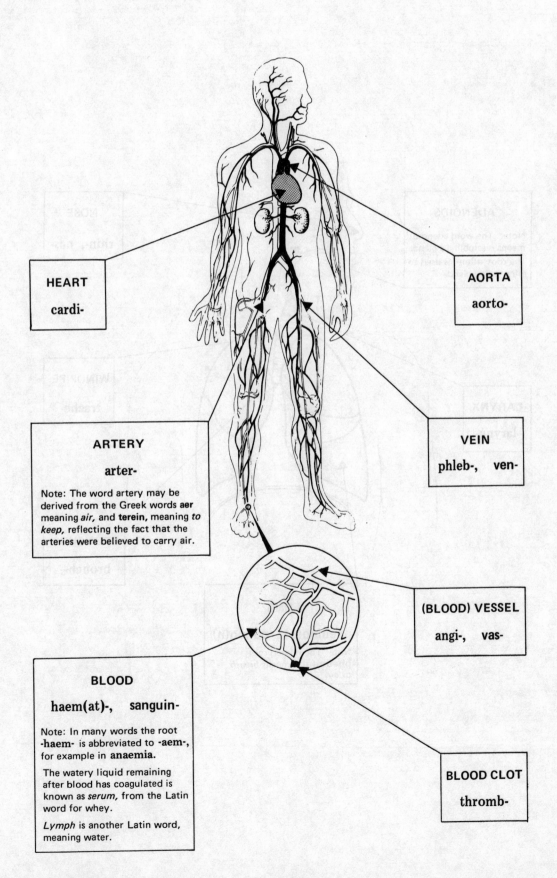

HEART

cardi-

AORTA

aorto-

ARTERY

arter-

Note: The word artery may be derived from the Greek words **aer** meaning *air,* and **terein,** meaning *to keep,* reflecting the fact that the arteries were believed to carry air.

VEIN

phleb-,   ven-

(BLOOD) VESSEL

angi-,   vas-

BLOOD

haem(at)-,   sanguin-

Note: In many words the root -haem- is abbreviated to -aem-, for example in **anaemia.**

The watery liquid remaining after blood has coagulated is known as *serum,* from the Latin word for whey.

Lymph is another Latin word, meaning water.

BLOOD CLOT

thromb-

THE RESPIRATORY SYSTEM

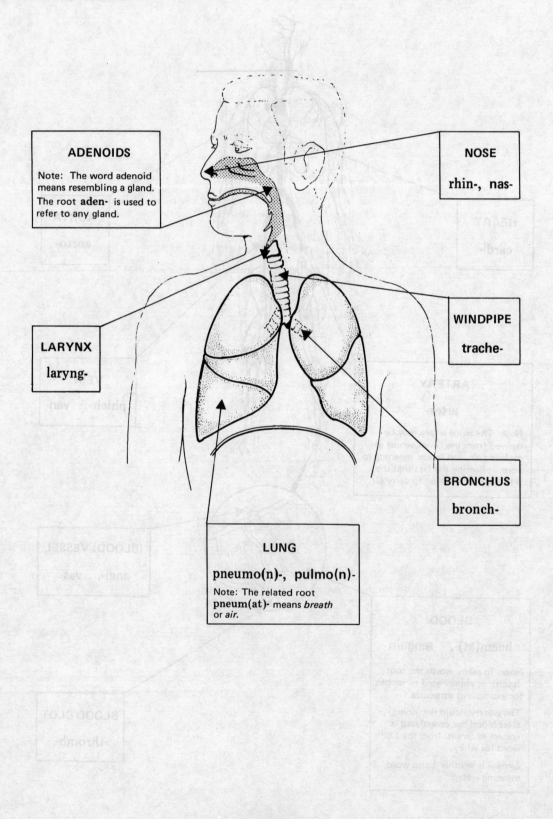

ADENOIDS

Note: The word adenoid means resembling a gland. The root **aden-** is used to refer to any gland.

NOSE

rhin-, nas-

LARYNX

laryng-

WINDPIPE

trache-

BRONCHUS

bronch-

LUNG

pneumo(n)-, pulmo(n)-

Note: The related root **pneum(at)-** means *breath* or *air*.

TEST

19. Which parts of the body are affected in the following diseases?

(a) Arteriosclerosis

(b) Phlebitis

(c) Polycythaemia

(d) Pneumonia

(e) Pulmonary emphysema

(f) Adenofibrosis.

20. Deduce the meaning of the following terms:

(a) Cardiology

(b) Aortogram

(c) Haemotherapy

(d) Pneumatocardia

(e) Tracheal

(f) Adenoneural

(g) Thrombus.

26

ANSWERS TO TEST

19. (a) Arteries
     (b) Veins
     (c) The blood
     (d) The lungs
     (e) The lungs
     (f) A gland.

20. (a) The study of the heart
     (b) A record of the aorta (produced by X-ray photography).
     (c) Treatment of disease with blood (or blood products)
     (d) The presence of air in the heart
     (e) Pertaining to the windpipe
     (f) Pertaining to a gland and a nerve
     (g) A blood clot.

THE URINARY SYSTEM

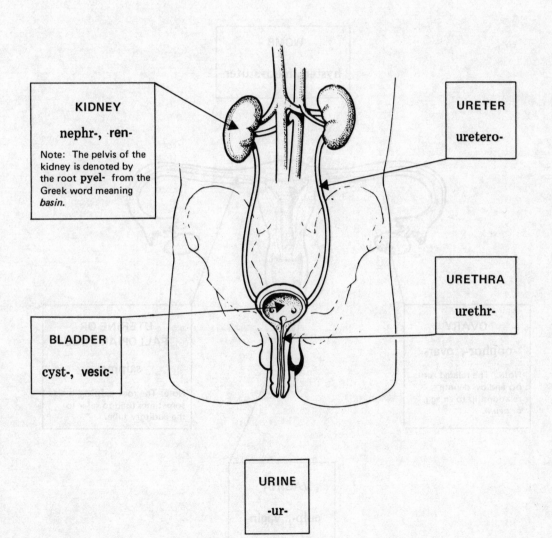

KIDNEY

nephr-, ren-

Note: The pelvis of the kidney is denoted by the root **pyel-** from the Greek word meaning *basin.*

URETER

uretero-

URETHRA

urethr-

BLADDER

cyst-, vesic-

URINE

-ur-

28

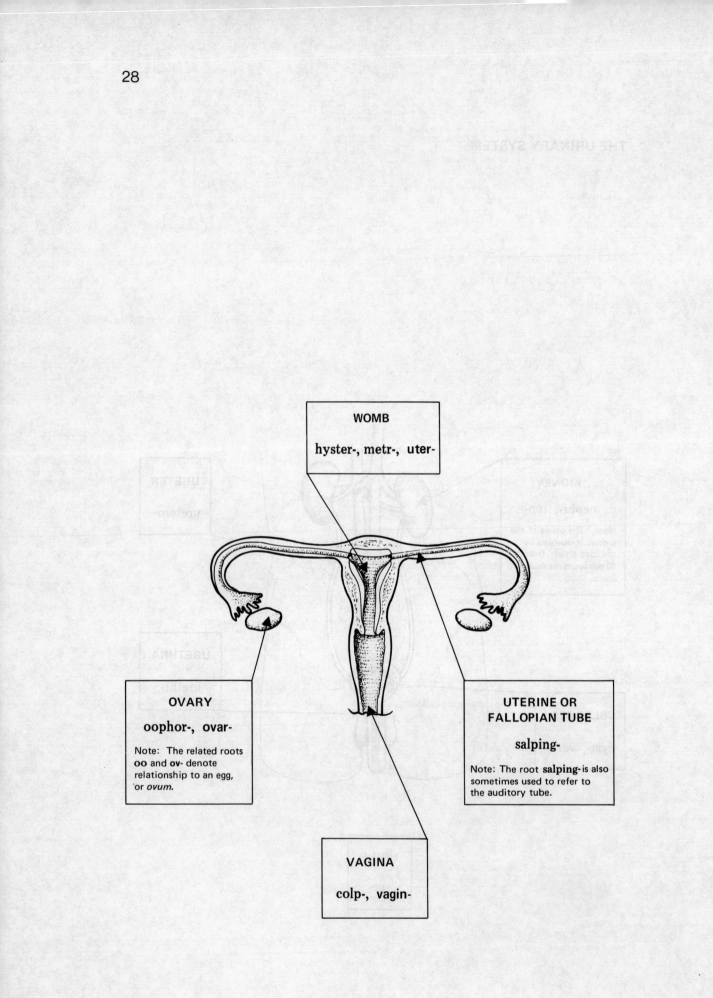

WOMB

hyster-, metr-, uter-

OVARY

oophor-, ovar-

Note: The related roots
oo and ov- denote
relationship to an egg,
or *ovum*.

UTERINE OR
FALLOPIAN TUBE

salping-

Note: The root salping- is also
sometimes used to refer to
the auditory tube.

VAGINA

colp-, vagin-

TEST

21. Deduce the meaning of the following terms:

    (a)   Haematuria

    (b)   Colpomicroscope

    (c)   Renal artery

    (d)   Pyelogram

    (e)   Nephrology

    (f)   Ovarian.

22. Which parts of the body are affected by the following diseases?

    (a)   Cystitis

    (b)   Endometriosis

    (c)   Pyelonephritis

    (d)   Salpingitis

    (e)   Urethritis.

23. On which parts of the body are the following surgical procedures carried out?

    (a)   Hysterectomy

    (b)   Vesicofixation

    (c)   Ureterostomy

    (d)   Oophoropexy

    (e)   Ovariotomy

ANSWERS TO TEST

21.   (a)   Blood in the urine

      (b)   A microscope used in the vagina

      (c)   An artery which supplies a kidney

      (d)   A record of the pelvis of the kidney (produced by X-ray photography)

      (e)   The study of the kidney

      (f)   Pertaining to the ovary.

22.   (a)   The bladder

      (b)   The womb

      (c)   The kidney

      (d)   The uterine tube or the auditory tube

      (e)   The urethra.

23.   (a)   The womb

      (b)   The bladder

      (c)   The ureter

      (d)   The ovary

      (e)   The ovary.

THE DIGESTIVE SYSTEM

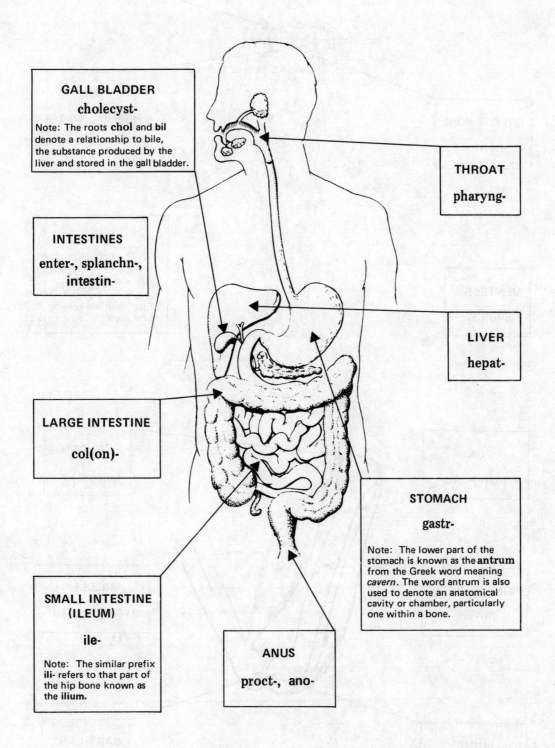

GALL BLADDER

cholecyst-

Note: The roots **chol** and **bil** denote a relationship to bile, the substance produced by the liver and stored in the gall bladder.

INTESTINES

enter-, splanchn-, intestin-

LARGE INTESTINE

col(on)-

SMALL INTESTINE (ILEUM)

ile-

Note: The similar prefix **ili-** refers to that part of the hip bone known as the **ilium.**

ANUS

proct-, ano-

THROAT

pharyng-

LIVER

hepat-

STOMACH

gastr-

Note: The lower part of the stomach is known as the **antrum** from the Greek word meaning *cavern*. The word antrum is also used to denote an anatomical cavity or chamber, particularly one within a bone.

THE LOCOMOTOR SYSTEM

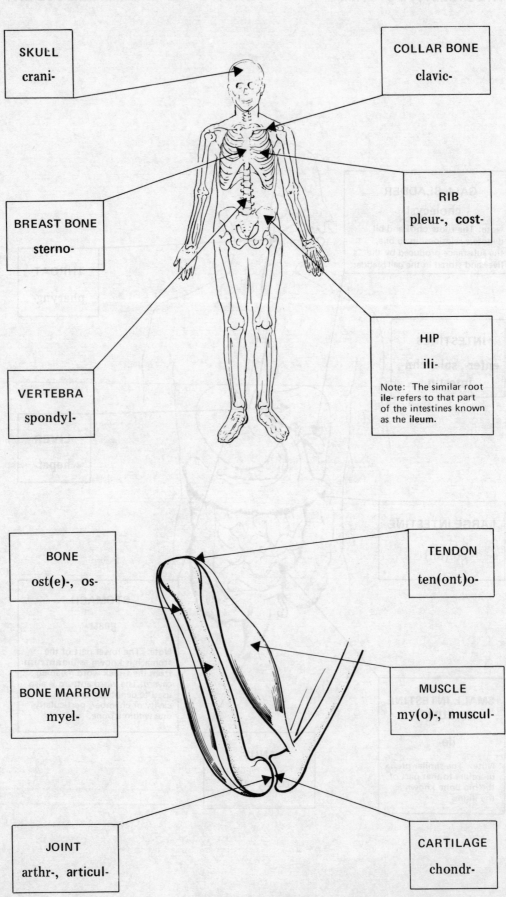

SKULL

crani-

COLLAR BONE

clavic-

BREAST BONE

sterno-

RIB

pleur-, cost-

VERTEBRA

spondyl-

HIP

ili-

Note: The similar root ile- refers to that part of the intestines known as the ileum.

BONE

ost(e)-, os-

TENDON

ten(ont)o-

BONE MARROW

myel-

MUSCLE

my(o)-, muscul-

JOINT

arthr-, articul-

CARTILAGE

chondr-

TEST

24. Which parts of the body are affected by the following diseases?

    (a) Osteitis

    (b) Hepatitis

    (c) Ankylosing spondylitis

    (d) Dysentery

    (e) Proctitis

    (f) Osteomyelitis.

25. Deduce which of the words on the left have the meanings listed on the right

(a) Chondrocyte	(i)	Removal of the stomach or part of the stomach
(b) Myelogram	(ii)	A record of types of cells found in a preparation of bone marrow
(c) Gastrectomy		
(d) Myogram	(iii)	A surgical incision of the colon in the region of the crest of the hip
(e) Iliocolotomy		
(f) Ileostomy	(iv)	Surgical procedure in which an opening into the small intestine is made
	(v)	A cartilage cell
	(vi)	A record of a muscular contraction

26. (a) Between which organs does the entero-hepatic circulation take place?

    (b) What region of the body is supplied by the splanchnic nerves?

    (c) Which two of the following words are synonyms (have the same meaning ?

        biliary,   intestinal,   colonic,   arthritis,   hepatic,   enteric.

34

CELLS AND TISSUES

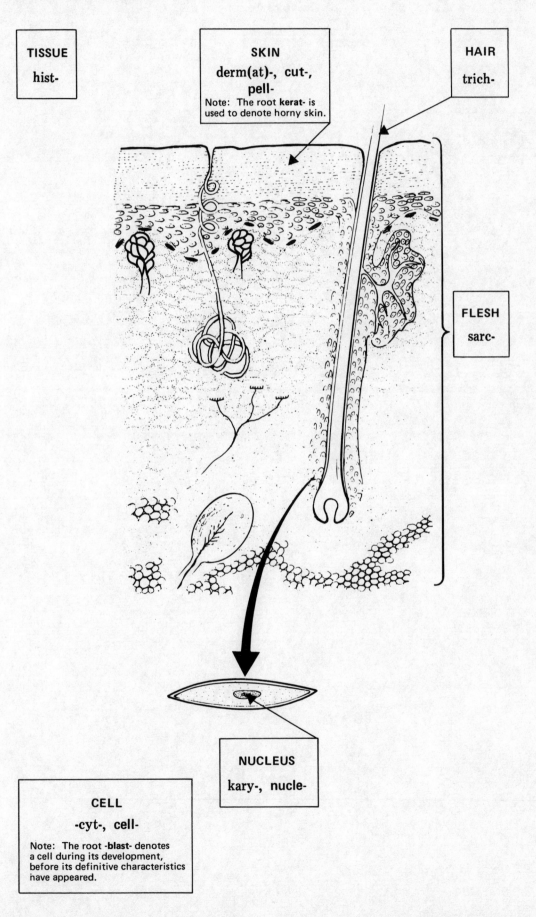

TISSUE
hist-

SKIN
derm(at)-, cut-, pell-
Note: The root **kerat-** is used to denote horny skin.

HAIR
trich-

FLESH
sarc-

NUCLEUS
kary-, nucle-

CELL
-cyt-, cell-
Note: The root **-blast-** denotes a cell during its development, before its definitive characteristics have appeared.

35

TEST

27. (a) What is histology?

(b) What feature would you expect to be prominent in the micro-organism *Trichomonas?*

(c) In the development of white blood cells which stage appears first, the lymphoblast or the lymphocyte?

(d) What is a karyocyte?

28. What parts of the body are affected by the following diseases?

(a) Pellagra

(b) Dermatitis

(c) Cutitis

(d) Sarcostosis.

ANSWERS TO TEST

27. (a) The study of tissues
     (b) They have hair-like projections (or flagella)
     (c) The lymphoblast
     (d) A cell with a nucleus.

28. (a) The skin (and also the alimentary tract and nervous system)
     (b) The skin
     (c) The skin
     (d) The fleshy tissues.

SENSES

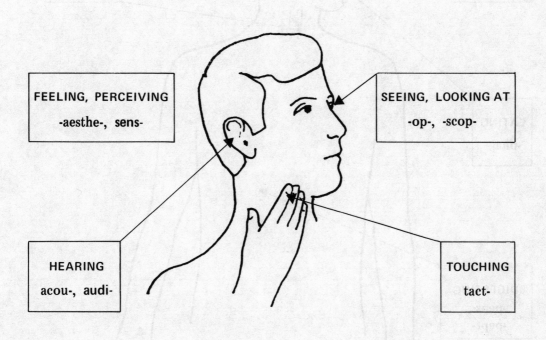

OTHER BODILY ACTIVITIES

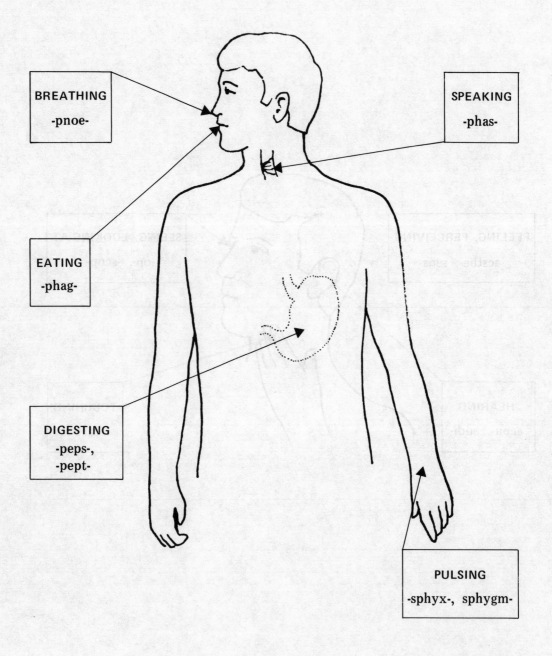

Other common roots associated with actions of the body are

cine- or kine	meaning *move*
par(t)-	meaning *to give birth*
-gen-	meaning *to cause* or *be caused, to produce* or *be produced, to become, to originate* or *be originated.*

TEST

29. Which of the definitions on the right apply to the words listed on the left?

(a) Phagocyte   (i) Pertaining to the sense of hearing

(b) Pepsin   (ii) Producing sensation

(c) Acoustic   (iii) An enzyme secreted by the stomach which digests proteins

(d) Otoscope

(e) Aesthesiogenic   (iv) A cell that ingests foreign particles

       (v) An instrument for inspecting the ear.

30. Deduce the meaning of the following words:

(a) Tactile

(b) Apnoea

(c) Dysphagia

(d) Anaesthesia

(e) Kinetic

(f) Dyspnoea

(g) Asphyxia

(**A**- or **an**- is a negative prefix; the prefix **dys**- means *difficulty*).

31. Which parts of the body are supplied by the following nerves?

(a) Optic nerve

(b) Auditory nerve

(c) Sensory nerves.

32. What sort of woman is nulliparous?

(**null** − means *none*).

42

Part three-Prepositions

There are a large number of prefixes of Greek and Latin origin which acts as prepositions when they are placed in front of a root word. (A preposition is a word which expresses a relation between the noun it governs and another word. Examples are *at, in, by, to, for, under.*) A single root can be modified to several words of different meaning by such prefixes.

For example

Prefix	Meaning	Root	Meaning	Word	Meaning
–	–	cardi	*heart*	–	–
ante-	*before*	cardi	*heart*	antecardium	The upper middle region of the abdomen before or against the heart
anti-	*against*	cardi	*heart*	anticardium	
dextr-	*to the right*	cardi	*heart*	dextrocardia	Location of the heart on the right side of the chest
endo-	*inside*	cardi	*heart*	endocardial	Situated or occurring within the heart
				endocardium	The innermost layer of the three layers of the heart wall
exo-	*outside*	cardi	*heart*	exocardial	Situated or occurring outside the heart
meso-	*middle*	cardi	*heart*	mesocardium	The middle layer of the three layers of the heart wall
peri-	*around*	cardi	*heart*	pericardium	The outer layer of the heart wall, a tissue which surrounds the heart
pre-	*before*	cardi	*heart*	precardiac	Situated before the heart
retro-	*backwards*	cardi	*heart*	retrocardiac	Situated behind the heart

44

IN, OUT, TO, FROM

OUT

ec-, ex-, e-

Note: The x of ex- is changed
to f before roots beginning
with f.

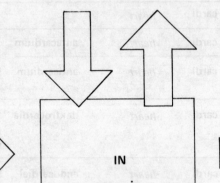

IN

en-, in-

Note: The n of en- is
changed to m before roots
beginning with the letters
b, p, or ph.

The n of in- is changed to
l, m, or r before roots
beginning with these
letters.

TOWARDS (NEAR)

ad-

Note: The d of ad- is changed
to c, f, g, p, s or t before
roots beginning with these
letters. (So the prefixes
ac-, af-, ag-, ap-, as- and **at-**
all mean *to*.

AWAY FROM (SEPARATE)

apo-, ab-

Note: The o of apo- is
dropped before roots
beginning with a vowel.

TEST

33. Match the correct meanings with the appropriate words, for each of the sets of words and meanings below.

(a)	Abduct	To draw away from
	Adduct	To draw towards
(b)	Afferent	Conducting outwards
	Efferent	Conducting towards
(c)	Expire	To breathe in
	Inspire	To breathe out
(d)	Eccrine	Secreting outwards
	Apocrine	Secreting when part of the secreting cell separates.

34. (a) Where would you expect to find the adrenal glands?

(b) Does an abnerval electric current pass towards or away from a nerve?

(c) What does adoral mean?

(d) What is the meaning and derivation of the prefix **encephalo-**?

35. Which of the definitions on the right apply to the words listed on the left?

(a)	Inferent	(i)	To cut out
(b)	Inversion	(ii)	Protrusion of the eyeball
(c)	Exophthalmos	(iii)	To make a cut in
(d)	Encolpism	(iv)	A turning outwards
(e)	Excise	(v)	Afferent
(f)	Eversion	(vi)	Medication by vaginal injections
(g)	Incise	(vii)	A turning inwards.

46

```
┌─────────────────────────────────────────────────────────────────────────┐
│ ANSWERS TO TEST                                                           │
│ 33.   (a)  Abduct      —  To draw away from                               │
│            Adduct      —  To draw towards                                 │
│                                                                           │
│       (b)  Afferent    —  Conducting towards                              │
│            Efferent    —  Conducting outwards                             │
│                                                                           │
│       (c)  Expire      —  To breathe out                                  │
│            Inspire     —  To breathe in                                   │
│                                                                           │
│       (d)  Eccrine     —  Secreting outwards                              │
│            Apocrine    —  Secreting when part of the secreting cell       │
│                           separates.                                      │
│                                                                           │
│ 34.   (a)  Near the kidneys                                               │
│       (b)  Away from                                                      │
│       (c)  Towards or near the mouth                                      │
│       (d)  Encephalo- means brain, from en-, meaning in, and cephalo-,    │
│            meaning skull.                                                 │
│                                                                           │
│ 35.   (a)                    (v)                                          │
│       (b)                    (vii)                                        │
│       (c)                    (ii)                                         │
│       (d)                    (vi)                                         │
│       (e)                    (i)                                          │
│       (f)                    (iv)                                         │
│       (g)                    (iii)                                        │
└─────────────────────────────────────────────────────────────────────────┘
```

INSIDE AND OUTSIDE, ABOVE AND BELOW

BEYOND (EXTREME)

ultra-

ABOVE

hyper-, super-, supra-

Note: **Hyper-** is usually used to mean above in the sense of too many or excessive.

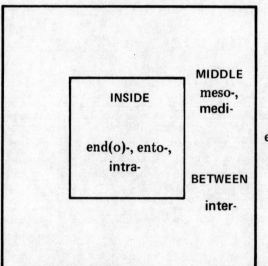

MIDDLE
meso-,
medi-

INSIDE

end(o)-, ento-,
intra-

BETWEEN

inter-

OUTSIDE
ect-, exo-, extra-

BELOW

hypo-, sub-

Note: **Hypo-** is usually used to mean below in the sense of too few or lack of.

The o of hypo- is dropped before roots beginning with a vowel.

The b of sub- is changed to f or p before roots beginning with these letters.

BENEATH

infra-

48

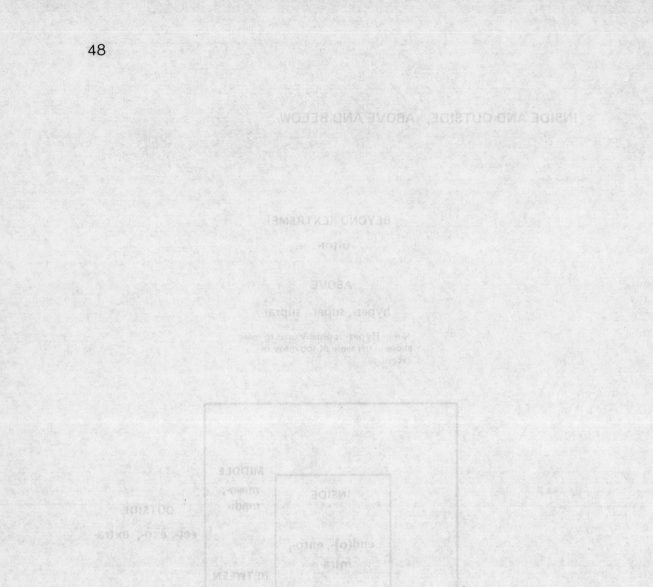

TEST

36. (a) The developing embryo consists of three layers of tissue, the ectoderm, the endoderm or entoderm, and the mesoderm. Which of these is
(i) the outermost layer (ii) the innermost layer?

(b) (i) Is a sweat gland an endocrine or an exocrine gland?
(ii) Are the adrenal glands endocrine or exocrine glands?
(iii) Are the salivary glands endocrine glands or exocrine glands?

37. Deduce the meaning of the following terms:
(a) Endoscope
(b) Mesonasal
(c) Interarticular
(d) Ectoparasite
(e) Medial.

38. Which of the definitions on the right apply to the terms listed on the left?
(a) Intracellular   (i) Situated between blood vessels
(b) Intercellular   (ii) Situated outside cells
(c) Extracellular   (iii) Situated between cells
(d) Intravascular   (iv) Situated within blood vessels
(e) Intervascular   (v) Situated outside blood vessels
(f) Extravascular   (vi) Situated within cells.

39. Where are the following sites?
(a) Suprahepatic
(b) Subclavicular
(c) Infrasternal
(d) Hypoglossal
(e) Infratracheal
(f) Supraocular
(g) Subcutaneous.

40. Which of the definitions on the right apply to the terms listed on the left?
(a) Hyperacusis   (i) Abnormally increased sugar content in the blood
(b) Hyperglycaemia
(c) Hypodermic   (ii) Low blood pressure
(d) Hypertension   (iii) High blood pressure
(e) Hypoglycaemia   (iv) Abnormally low sugar content in the blood
(f) Hypotension   (v) Abnormal acuteness of the sense of hearing
                      (vi) Applied beneath the skin.

ANSWERS TO TEST

36. (a) (i)   Ectoderm
        (ii) Endoderm or entoderm

    (b) (i)   Exocrine
        (ii) Endocrine
        (iii) Exocrine.

37. (a) An instrument for viewing internal parts of the body.
    (b) In the middle of the nose.
    (c) Between the surfaces of a joint.
    (d) A parasite which lives on the outside of its host.
    (e) Pertaining to the middle.

38. (a)   (vi)
    (b)   (iii)
    (c)   (ii)
    (d)   (iv)
    (e)   (i)
    (f)   (v)

39. (a) Above the liver.
    (b) Under the collar bone.
    (c) Beneath the breast bone.
    (d) Under the tongue.
    (e) Beneath the windpipe
    (f) Above the eye.
    (g) Under the skin.

40. (a)   (v)
    (b)   (i)
    (c)   (vi)
    (d)   (iii)
    (e)   (iv)
    (f)   (ii)

TOGETHER, APART, THROUGH, ROUND

WITH, TOGETHER

syn-, con-

Note: The n of syn is changed to l before the letter l,

to m before the letters b, m, p, and ph, and is dropped before the letter s.

The n of con- is changed to l before the letter l, to m before the letters b, m and p, to r before the letter r, and is dropped before h, and vowels.

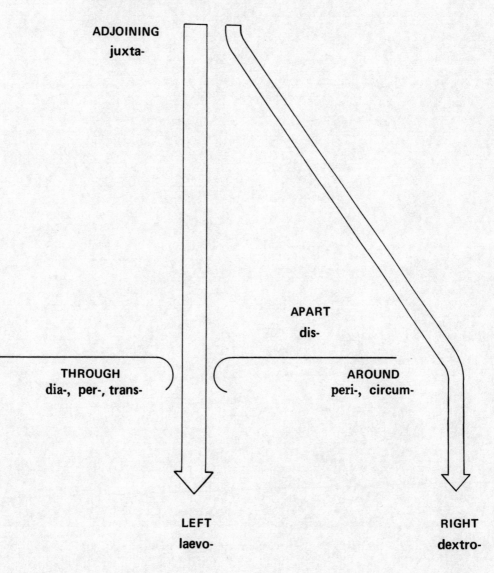

ADJOINING
juxta-

APART
dis-

THROUGH
dia-, per-, trans-

AROUND
peri-, circum-

LEFT
laevo-

RIGHT
dextro-

TEST

41. Which is the correct word of the alternatives given in the sentences below?
  (a) During diastole the walls of the heart are together/apart.
  (b) During systole the walls of the heart are together/apart.
  (c) Dextromanual means left-/right- handed.
  (d) To dissect is to cut apart/through.
  (e) The fibres of a muscle that contracts are drawn apart/together.

42. Deduce the meanings of the following terms.
  (a) Contact
  (b) Periosteum
  (c) Per os
  (d) Circumintestinal
  (e) Transdermic
  (f) Percutaneous.

43. Deduce which of the definitions on the right apply to the terms listed on the left.
  (a) Peritoneum
  (b) Symbiotic
  (c) Juxtaposed
  (d) Diathermy

  (i) Living together
  (ii) Placed side by side.
  (iii) The generation of heat in tissues due to passage of an electric current through them.
  (iv) The membrane which is stretched around the inside of the abdominal cavity and lines it.

54

ANSWERS TO TEST

41. (a) apart
   (b) together
   (c) right
   (d) apart
   (e) together.

42. (a) Touch together
   (b) A tissue which covers bones
   (c) Through the mouth
   (d) Around the intestines
   (e) (Passed) through the skin
   (f) (Performed) through the skin.

43. (a)   (iv)
   (b)   (i)
   (c)   (ii)
   (d)   (iii)

UP, DOWN, BACK, AGAINST

UP (POSITIVE)

ana-

Note: The second a of ana- is dropped before roots beginning with a vowel.

DOWN (NEGATIVE)

cata-, de-

Note: The second a of cata- is dropped before roots beginning with a vowel.

BACK (AGAIN)

re-

BACKWARDS

opistho-, retr-

AGAINST

anti-, contra-

Note: The i of anti- is dropped before roots beginning with a vowel.

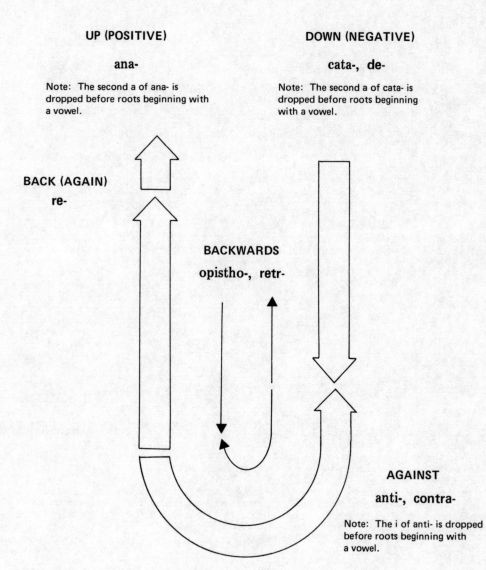

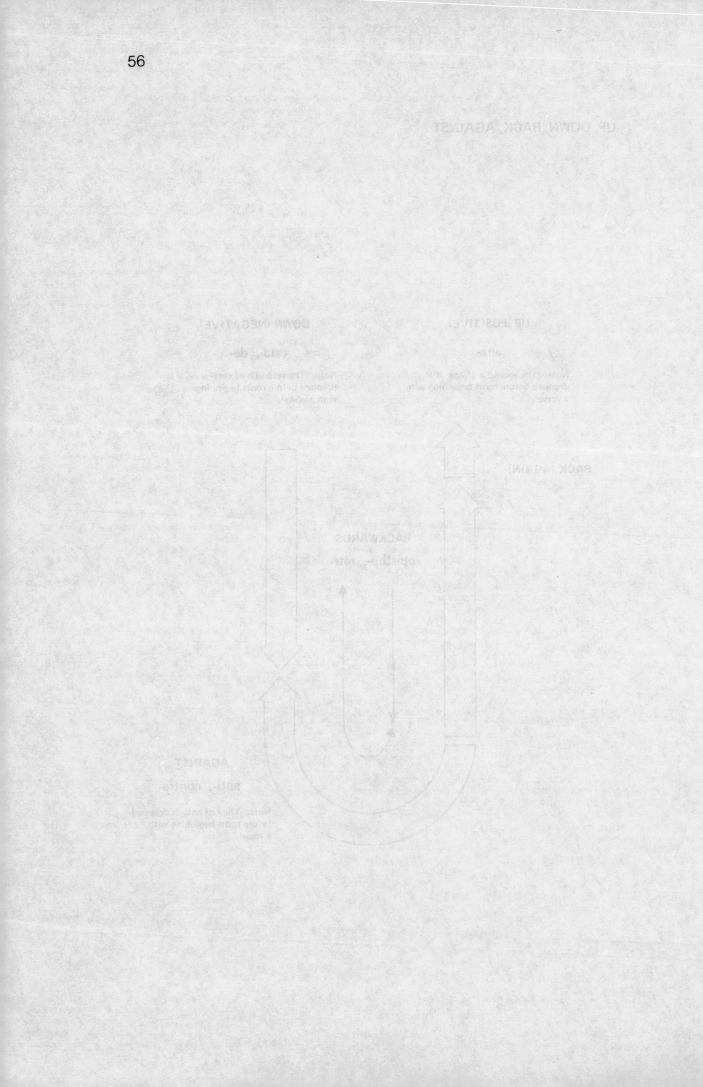

TEST

44. Match the correct meanings with the appropriate words for each of the sets of words and meanings below.

(a) Anabolism — Breaking down of complex substances in body tissues into simpler substances.

Catabolism — Building up of complex substances in body tissues from simpler substances.

(b) Opisthencephalon — The cerebellum, which lies below and behind the main part of the brain.

Opisthotonos — A form of muscle spasm in which the head and legs are bent backwards.

(c) Retrobuccal — Behind the tongue.

Retrolingual — Pertaining to the back of the mouth.

(d) Depression — State of sadness, feeling of hopelessness, of being 'pressed down'.

Repression — The 'pressing back' into the unconscious of conscious ideas of a disagreeable nature.

45. Deduce the meaning of the following terms:

(a) Decapitate

(b) Contraindication

(c) Retrocolic

(d) Antihyperglycaemic.

ANSWERS TO TEST

44.

(a) Anabolism — Building up of complex substances in body tissues from simpler substances.

Catabolism — Breaking down of complex substances in body tissues into simpler substances.

(b) Opisthencephalon — The cerebellum, which lies below and behind the main part of the brain.

Opisthotonos — A form of muscle spasm in which the head and legs are bent backwards.

(c) Retrobuccal — Pertaining to the back part of the mouth.

Retrolingual — Behind the tongue.

(d) Depression — State of sadness, feeling of hopelessness, of being 'pressed down'.

Repression — The 'pressing back' into the unconscious of conscious ideas of a disagreeable nature.

45.

(a) Remove the head.

(b) An indication against (for example, against the use of a particular treatment).

(c) Behind the colon.

(d) Countering high levels of sugar in the blood.

UPON, BEFORE, BEHIND, BACK, SIDE

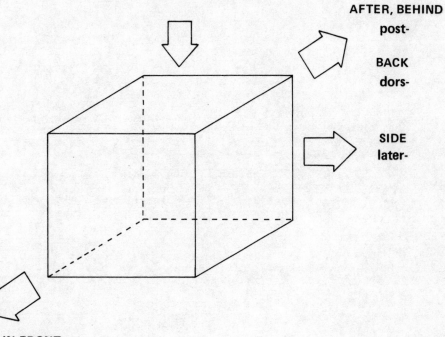

UPON (IN ADDITION, AFTER)

epi-

Note: The i of epi- is dropped before roots beginning with a vowel.

AFTER, BEHIND
post-

BACK
dors-

SIDE
later-

BEFORE, IN FRONT
pro-, ante-, pre-, ventr-

Two other common prepositional prefixes are **meta-** and **para-**. **Meta-** can mean *next to* or *after,* as in metacarpals (the bones next to the wrist bones). **Para-** can mean *beside* or *beyond,* as in parathyroid (a gland beside the thyroid). However, both prefixes are also used to denote a change or modification as in met(a)haemoglobin (changed haemoglobin), metamorphosis (change in shape), paraesthesia (change in sensation), and paratyphoid (a modified form of typhoid).

TEST

46. Deduce the meaning of the following terms:

(a) Epidermis

(b) Procephalic

(c) Dorsointercostal

(d) Postmalarial

(e) Posthepatic

(f) Preauricular

(g) Prepartal.

47. From the following list of words select pairs which mean the same:

(a) Adrenal

(b) Ventral

(c) Forearm

(d) Anterior

(e) Dorsal

(f) Epinephros

(g) Antebrachium

(h) Posterior.

ANSWERS TO TEST

46. (a) The outermost layer of skin

(b) Situated at the front of the head

(c) Situated in the back and between the ribs

(d) Occurring after malaria

(e) Situated behind the liver

(f) Situated in front of the ear

(g) Occurring before childbirth.

47. (a)   (f)

(b)   (d)

(c)   (g)

(e)   (h).

ANATOMICAL PLANES AND POSITIONS

Some of the prefixes considered earlier in this section occur in the terms used to describe the location and relations of parts of the body.

The body is studied from the so-called *anatomical position* in which it stands upright with the feet together and parallel, with the arms by the sides and palms of the hands facing forwards, and with the head erect and eyes looking forwards.

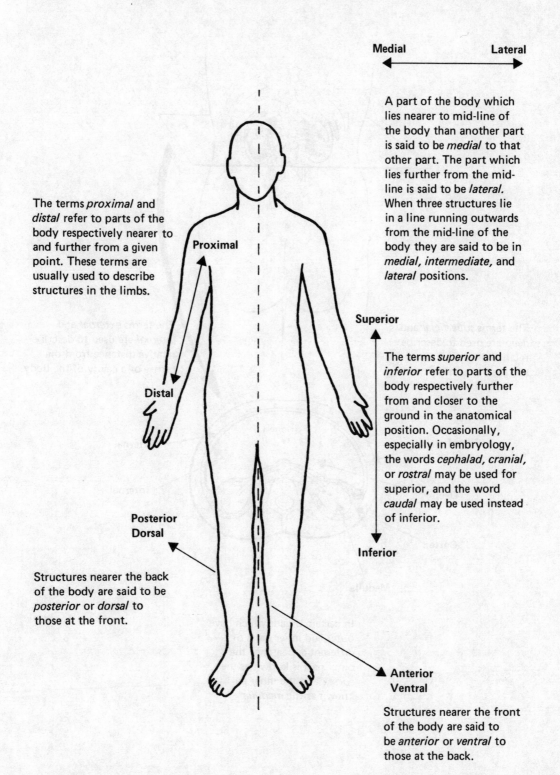

Medial ←——→ **Lateral**

A part of the body which lies nearer to mid-line of the body than another part is said to be *medial* to that other part. The part which lies further from the mid-line is said to be *lateral.* When three structures lie in a line running outwards from the mid-line of the body they are said to be in *medial, intermediate,* and *lateral* positions.

The terms *proximal* and *distal* refer to parts of the body respectively nearer to and further from a given point. These terms are usually used to describe structures in the limbs.

Proximal

Distal

Superior

The terms *superior* and *inferior* refer to parts of the body respectively further from and closer to the ground in the anatomical position. Occasionally, especially in embryology, the words *cephalad, cranial,* or *rostral* may be used for superior, and the word *caudal* may be used instead of inferior.

Inferior

Posterior Dorsal

Structures nearer the back of the body are said to be *posterior* or *dorsal* to those at the front.

Anterior Ventral

Structures nearer the front of the body are said to be *anterior* or *ventral* to those at the back.

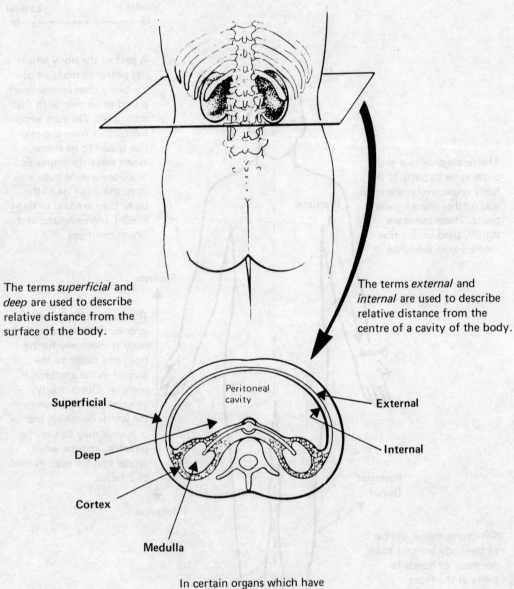

The terms *superficial* and *deep* are used to describe relative distance from the surface of the body.

The terms *external* and *internal* are used to describe relative distance from the centre of a cavity of the body.

Peritoneal cavity

Superficial

External

Deep

Internal

Cortex

Medulla

In certain organs which have outer and inner parts of different appearance the outer part is known as the *cortex* and the inner part is known as the *medulla*.

The various parts of the body may be described in relation to sections made through the body in different planes.

A section exactly in the mid-line at right angles to the coronal plane is said to be in the *median sagittal plane.* Any section parallel to this is known as a *sagittal* or *parasagittal section.*

A section through the body from side to side dividing the body into anterior and posterior portions is said to be in the *coronal plane* or *frontal plane.*

A section through the body dividing it into upper and lower parts is said to be in a *horizontal* or *transverse plane.*

TEST

48. (a) The diagram alongside shows the
left knee viewed from the rear.
Label (i) the medial ligament
(ii) the lateral ligament.

(b) The diagram alongside shows the
heart and the two largest veins
which enter it.
Label (i) the inferior vena cava
(ii) the superior vena cava.

(c) The diagram alongside shows the
bones of the hand. Which of the
phalanges indicated are
(i) proximal to the wrist
(ii) distal to the wrist?

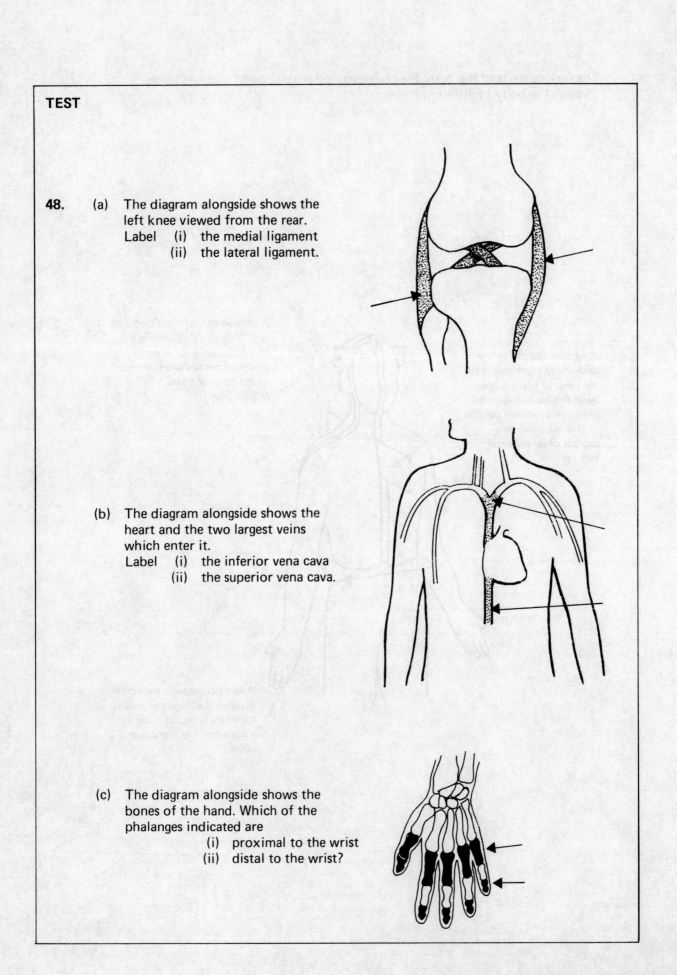

(d) The diagram alongside shows some
of the arteries of the left leg. Which
of the arteries indicated is
 (i) the posterior tibial artery
 (ii) the anterior tibial artery.

49. (a) On the diagrams shown alongside
label (i) the external iliac artery
 (ii) the internal iliac artery

(b) Which of the definitions on the right apply to the terms on the left:

(a) Superficial   (i)   Situated towards the front of the body

(b) Dorsal   (ii)   Situated far beneath the surface of
 the body

(c) Ventral   (iii)

(d) Deep   (iii)   Situated near the surface of the body

           (iv)   Anterior.

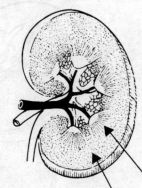

(c) The diagram alongside shows a
cross-section through the
kidney. Label:
 (i) the cortex
 (ii) the medulla.

50   In which planes have the following sections
      through the body been taken?

(a)

(b)

(c)

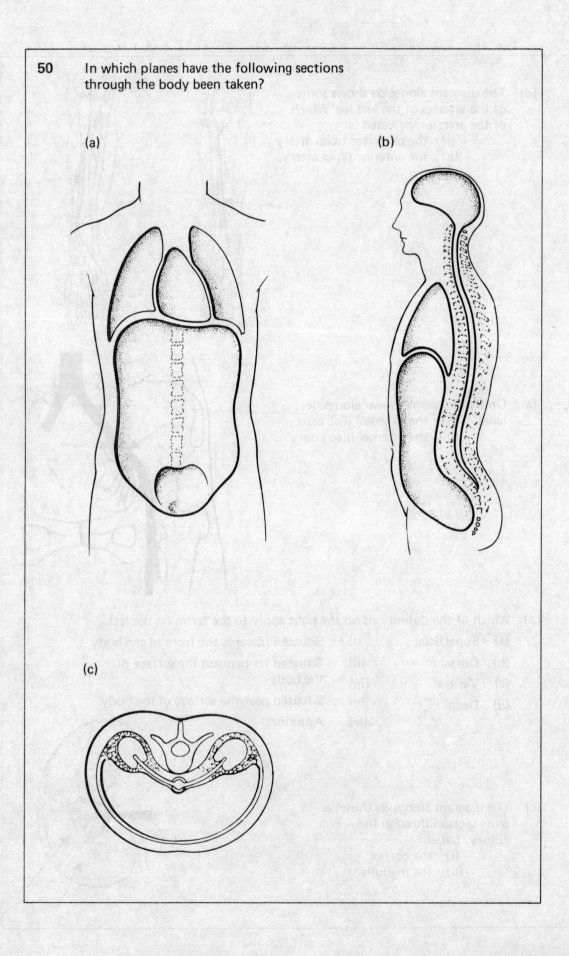

ANSWERS TO TEST
48.   (a)

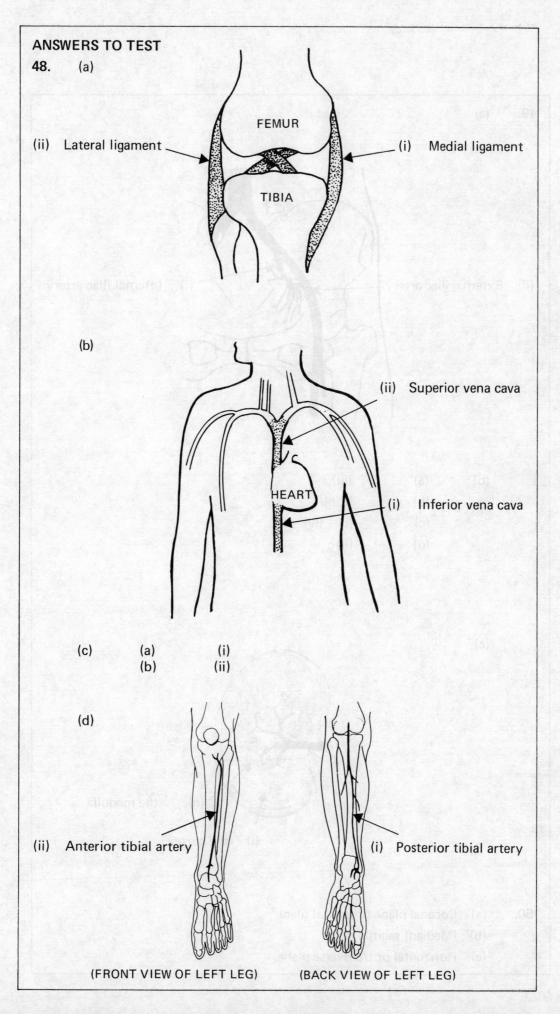

(ii) Lateral ligament   (i) Medial ligament

FEMUR

TIBIA

(b)

(ii) Superior vena cava

HEART

(i) Inferior vena cava

(c)   (a)   (i)
          (b)   (ii)

(d)

(ii) Anterior tibial artery   (i) Posterior tibial artery

(FRONT VIEW OF LEFT LEG)   (BACK VIEW OF LEFT LEG)

49. (a)

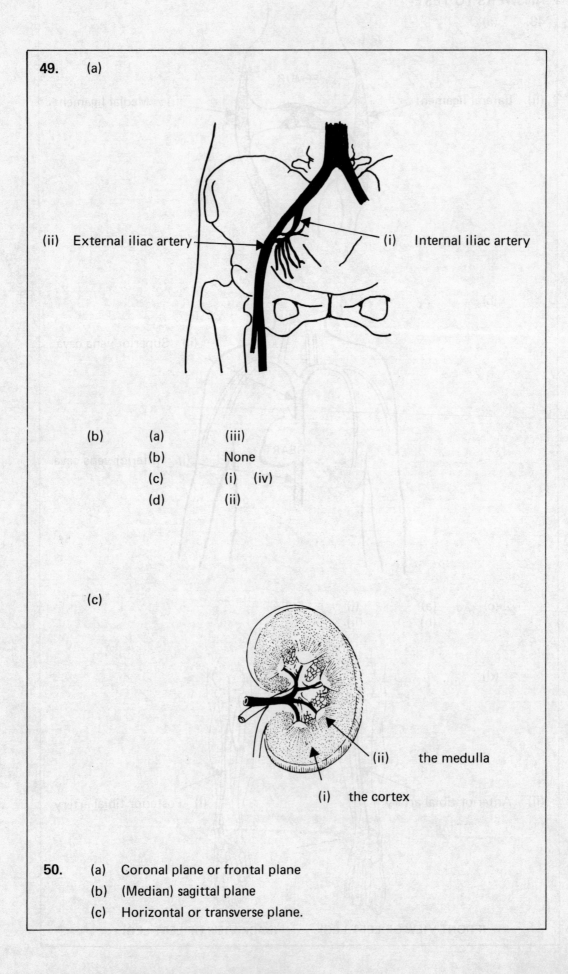

(ii) External iliac artery   (i)   Internal iliac artery

(b)   (a)   (iii)
          (b)   None
          (c)   (i)   (iv)
          (d)   (ii)

(c)

(ii)   the medulla

(i)   the cortex

50. (a) Coronal plane or frontal plane
      (b) (Median) sagittal plane
      (c) Horizontal or transverse plane.

Part four - Adjectives

QUANTITY

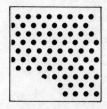

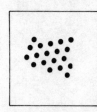

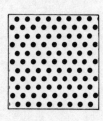

MANY (EXCESS)
poly-, hyper-, multi-

FEW (UNDER)
oligo-, hypo-,
-pen(ia)

ALL
pan-

NONE
a-, in

Note: a- becomes an- before
roots beginning with a vowel or h.
The n of in- changes to l before l,
to m before b, m and p, and to r
before r.

Both a- and in- can be used to mean
a complete absence or a relative
deficiency.

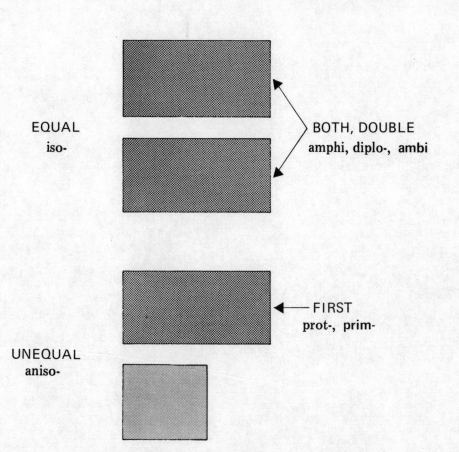

EQUAL
iso-

BOTH, DOUBLE
amphi, diplo-, ambi

FIRST
prot-, prim-

UNEQUAL
aniso-

TEST

51. Which of the definitions on the right apply to the words listed on the left?

(a) Anuria   (i) The passage of a large volume of urine

(b) Oliguria   (ii) Absence of excretion of urine from the body

(c) Polyuria   (iii) Excretion of a diminished amount of urine.

52. Deduce the meanings of the following words:

(a) Cytopenia

(b) Isodontic

(c) Protonephros

(d) Ambilateral

(e) Panmyelopathy

(f) Imbalance.

53. Match the correct meanings with the appropriate words for each of the sets of words and meanings below.

(a) Hypoaethesia   Abnormally increased sensitivity
    Hyperaesthesia   Abnormally decreased sensitivity

(b) Isopia   Double vision
    Anisopia   Equality of vision in the two eyes
    Diplopia   Inequality of vision in the two eyes

(c) Primiparous   Having borne one child
    Multiparous   Having borne two or more children.

74

ANSWERS TO TEST

51.   (a)   (ii)

       (b)   (iii)

       (c)   (i)

52.   (a) A lack of cells (in the blood)

       (b) Having teeth of the same size

       (c) The embryonic structure from which the kidney develops

       (d) Pertaining to both sides

       (e) A disease affecting all the bone marrow

       (f) Lack of balance.

53.   (a) Hypoaesthesia — Abnormally decreased sensitivity

           Hyperaesthesia — Abnormally increased sensitivity

       (b) Isopia — Equality of vision in the two eyes

           Anisopia — Inequality of vision in the two eyes

           Diplopia — Double vision

       (c) Primiparous — Having borne one child

           Multiparous — Having borne two or more children.

NUMBERS

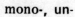 hemi-, semi

1 mono-, un-

2 di-, bi-

3 tri-, ter-

4 tetr-, quadr-

5 pent-, quinqu-

6 hex-, sex-

8 oct-

10 deca-, deci-

100 hect-, centi-

1 000 kilo-, milli-

1 000 000 mega-, micro-

The Greek and Latin prefixes for ten, hundred, thousand and million are used as prefixes for units in the metric system. Greek prefixes in this system denote *multiplied by;* Latin prefixes denote *divided by.* Therefore a kilometre is a thousand metres, whilst a millimetre is one-thousandth of a metre.

TEST

54. Place the following units of weight in ascending order of size:

(a) Milligram

(b) Kilogram

(c) Microgram

(d) Gram

(e) Centigram

(f) Hectogram

(g) Decigram.

55. Deduce the meaning of the following terms:

(a) Hemifacial

(b) Semicoma

(c) Megavolt

(d) Decalitre

(e) Monotic

(f) Unilateral.

56 Which of the definitions on the right apply to the terms listed on the left?

(a) Bipedal (i) A thing having three feet

(b) Hexadactylia (ii) Having only two fingers on one hand

(c) Tripod (iii) To cut into four parts

(d) Didactylous (iv) With both feet

(e) Quadrisect (v) Having six fingers on one hand.

78

SIZE AND SHAPE

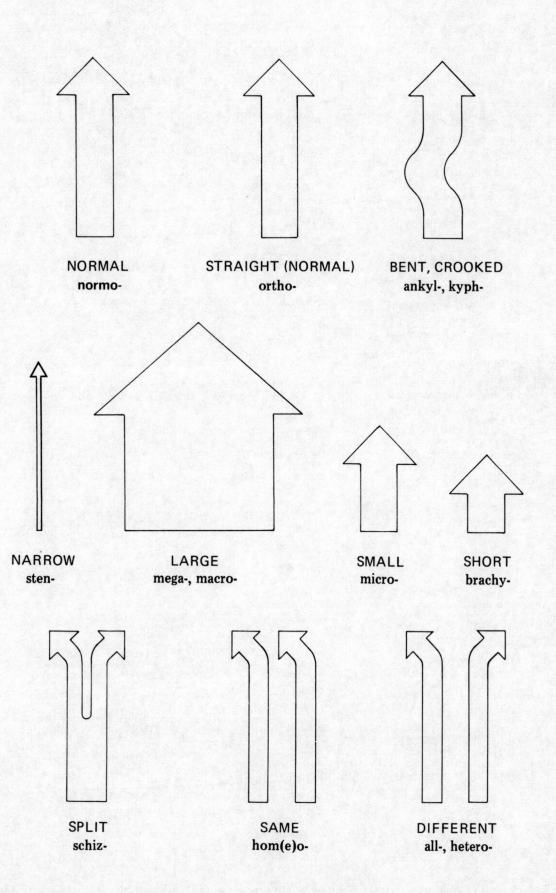

| NORMAL
normo- | STRAIGHT (NORMAL)
ortho- | BENT, CROOKED
ankyl-, kyph- |

| NARROW
sten- | LARGE
mega-, macro- | SMALL
micro- | SHORT
brachy- |

| SPLIT
schiz- | SAME
hom(e)o- | DIFFERENT
all-, hetero- |

80

TEST

57. Deduce the meaning of the following words

    (a) Stenocephalous

    (b) Megacolon

    (c) Brachyoesophagus

    (d) Schizophrenia

    (e) Normocyte

    (f) Microcheiria

    (g) Orthoglycaemic

58. Which of the definitions on the right apply to the terms listed on the left?

(a) Homogeneous	(i)	Formation of a stiff, often crooked, joint
(b) Heterogeneous	(ii)	Composed of ingredients of the same kind
(c) Macromastia	(iii)	Oversized breasts
(d) Allorhythmia	(iv)	Narrowed
(e) Stenosed	(v)	Irregularity of the heart beat
(f) Ankylosis	(vi)	Composed of different ingredients.

82

ANSWERS TO TEST

57.
  (a) Having a narrow head

  (b) An abnormally large colon

  (c) Abnormal shortness of the oesophagus

  (d) 'Split mind'. (Schizophrenia is a mental disorder in which there is disconnection between thoughts, feelings and actions.)

  (e) A (red blood) cell of normal size, shape and colour

  (f) Abnormal smallness of the hands

  (g) Having the normal amount of sugar in the blood.

58.
  (a)   (ii)

  (b)   (vi)

  (c)   (iii)

  (d)   (v)

  (e)   (iv)

  (f)   (i)

COLOUR
chrom-

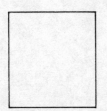

WHITE
leuc-, leuk-, alb-

BLACK (DARK)
melan-

GREY
polio-

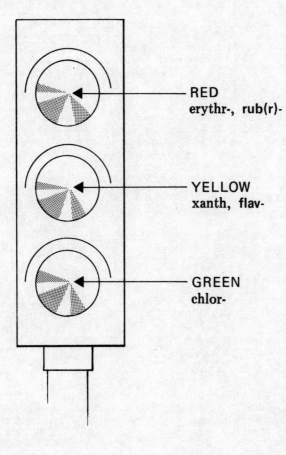

RED
erythr-, rub(r)-

YELLOW
xanth, flav-

BLUE
cyan-

GREEN
chlor-

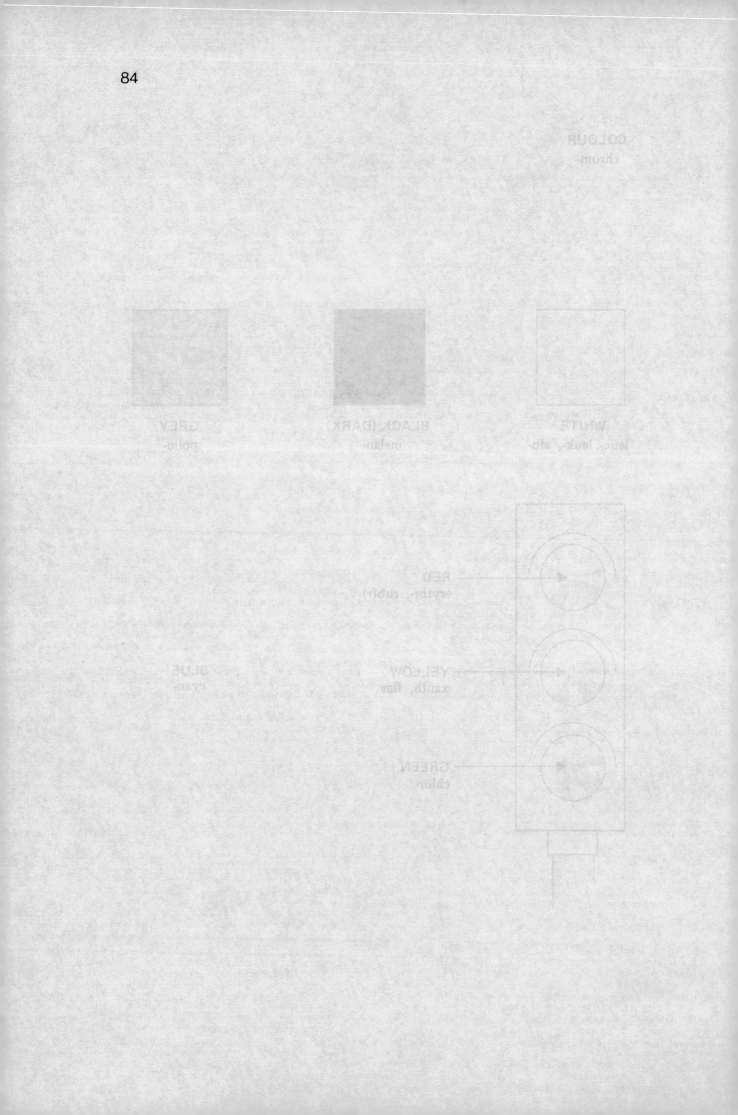

TEST

59. What colour are the following substances?

    (a)   Leucocytes

    (b)   Erythrocytes

    (c)   Chlorine

    (d)   Albumin

    (e)   Flavoxanthin.

60. Which of the definitions on the right apply to the terms listed on the left?

(a)	Chromocyte	(i)	Redness
(b)	Cyanosis	(ii)	A viral disease in which the *grey* matter of the nervous system is affected
(c)	Melanodermic		
(d)	Rubor	(iii)	A coloured cell
(e)	Poliomyelitis	(iv)	Having a black skin
		(v)	A bluish discoloration (particularly a discoloration of the skin and lips due to a reduction in the amount of oxygen in the blood).

ANSWERS TO TEST

59. (a) White

(b) Red

(c) Green

(d) White

(e) Yellow.

60. (a)   (iii)

(b)   (v)

(c)   (iv)

(d)   (i)

(e)   (ii).

SUBSTANCES

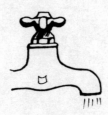
WATER
hydro-

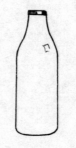
MILK
lact-

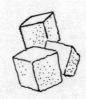
SUGAR (SWEET)
gluc-, glyc-, sacchar-

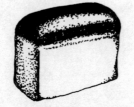
STARCH
amyl-

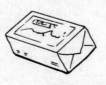
FAT
lip-, stear-, steat-, adip-

SODIUM Na
natr-

POTASSIUM K
kal-

STONE
-lith-, calc-

Certain suffixes are used to denote groups of substances. For example, the ending -**ose** indicates a *sugar,* as in glucose, lactose ('milk sugar') and maltose ('malt sugar'); and the ending -**ase** indicates an enzyme, as in lactase (the enzyme which catalyses the breakdown of lactose) and enterokinase.

Other common endings of this type are:

-**ide** — denoting derivatives of sugars, for example disacchar**ide**, glycos**ide**;

-**in** — used for various substances rather than substances of any specific type, for example peps**in** (an enzyme), glycer**in**;

-**ine** — often used for substances derived from (or once thought to be derived from) ammonia, for example am**ine**, chol**ine**;

-**ite** — often denotes end products, for example metabol**ite**;

-**gen** — often denotes a precursor, for example pepsino**gen** is the precursor of pepsin, being converted to pepsin by the action of hydrochloric acid.

TEST

61. Deduce the meaning of the following terms:

(a) Hydropenia

(b) Hypernatraemia

(c) Steatogenous

(d) Otoliths

(e) Kaliuresis

(f) Lipase.

62. Assign the substances listed below to the correct group by placing ticks in the appropriate boxes.

		Sugar	Sugar derivative	Enzyme	Precursor
(a)	Galactose	( )	( )	( )	( )
(b)	Amylase	( )	( )	( )	( )
(c)	Hydrolase	( )	( )	( )	( )
(d)	Fructoside	( )	( )	( )	( )
(e)	Trypsinogen	( )	( )	( )	( )

63. Define the following adjectives:

(a) Lactic

(b) Saccharine

(c) Amylogenic

(d) Adipose.

90

ANSWERS TO TEST

61.
(a) A deficiency of water (in the body)

(b) An excessive amount of sodium in the blood

(c) Producing fat

(d) 'Ear stones' (otoliths are crystals of calcium carbonate embedded in a gelatinous mass and found in certain sensory areas of the inner ear)

(e) The secretion of potassium in the urine

(f) An enzyme which breaks down fats.

62.

	Sugar	Sugar derivative	Enzyme	Precursor
(a)	(/)	( )	( )	( )
(b)	( )	( )	(/)	( )
(c)	( )	( )	(/)	( )
(d)	( )	(/)	( )	( )
(e)	( )	( )	( )	(/)

63.
(a) Pertaining to milk

(b) Sugary

(c) Producing starch

(d) Fatty.

HUMAN RELATIONS

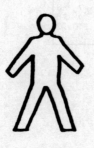

MALE
andr-

FEMALE
gyn(ec)-

CHILD
paed-

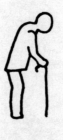

OLD MAN
ger(on)-

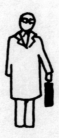

DOCTOR
-iatr-

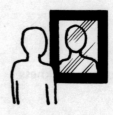

SELF
auto-

OTHER ADJECTIVAL PREFIXES

Time
chron-

NIGHT
nyct-, noct

MONTH
men-

Speed

FAST
tachy-

SLOW
brady-

Hardness, thickness

THICK
pachy-

HARD
scler-, dur-

TEST

64. Which of the definitions on the right apply to the terms listed on the left ?

(a)	Paediatric	(i)	Producing masculine characteristics
(b)	Androgenic	(ii)	Having both male and female characteristics
(c)	Gynecoid	(iii)	Pertaining to the treatment of disease in old people
(d)	Geriatric		
(e)	Gynandrism	(iv)	Resembling a woman
		(v)	Pertaining to the treatment of disease in children.

65.
(a) What is characteristic about autodermic grafts?

(b) Why are menstrual periods so called?

(c) When does nocturia occur?

(d) What, literally, is arteriosclerosis?

66. Deduce the meanings of the following terms.

(a) Bradycardia

(b) Tachycardia

(c) Pachyderma

(d) Autognosis.

94

ANSWERS TO TEST

64.   (a)   (v)

        (b)   (i)

        (c)   (iv)

        (d)   (iii)

        (e)   (ii)

65.   (a)   They are made of the patient's own skin

        (b)   Because they occur approximately monthly

        (c)   At night-time

        (d)   Hardening of the arteries.

66.   (a)   Slowness of the heart beat

        (b)   A fast heart rate

        (c)   (Abnormal) thickening of the skin

        (d)   Self-knowledge.

Part five-Disorder and disease

The names for many diseases and disease symptoms are simply expressed as deviations from normality using roots and prefixes already mentioned. For example:

ametria	–	absence of a uterus
bradypnoea	–	abnormally slow breathing
hypertrophy	–	excessive increase in size of an organ or part (from **hyper** and **trophe**, meaning *nutrition*)
hypocythaemia	–	deficiency of red cells in the blood
megaduodenum	–	abnormally large duodenum
polytrichia	–	excessive growth of hair.

Other prefixes used in naming diseases and symptoms in a similar way include the following:

dys-
mal- } meaning *bad, abnormal, painful* or *difficult*
(The opposite of dys- is **eu-** meaning *good* or *normal*. The opposite of mal- is **normo-**.)

atel-	meaning	*imperfect*
carcin-	meaning	*cancer*
pseud-	meaning	*false*
py-	meaning	*pus*
tox-	meaning	*poison*

TEST

67. Which of the definitions on the right apply to the terms listed on the left?

(a)	Atelopodia	(i)	Skin disease caused by a poison
(b)	Eupepsia	(ii)	Wasting caused by lack of nutrition
(c)	Atrophy	(iii)	An apparent loss of muscle power
(d)	Pyocolpos	(iv)	Hypertrophy of the heart
(e)	Pseudoparalysis	(v)	Normal digestion
(f)	Megalocardia	(vi)	Imperfect development of the foot
(g)	Toxicoderma	(vii)	A collection of pus in the vagina.

68. Deduce the meaning of the following terms.
(a) Dyspnoea
(b) Atelocephalous
(c) Toxaemia
(d) Carcinogenic
(e) Microstomia
(f) Atrichia
(g) Malabsorption.

96

ANSWERS TO TEST

67.　(a)　　　(vi)
　　(b)　　　(v)
　　(c)　　　(ii)
　　(d)　　　(vii)
　　(e)　　　(iii)
　　(f)　　　(iv)
　　(g)　　　(i)

68.　(a)　Difficult or painful breathing
　　(b)　Imperfect development of the head
　　(c)　Blood poisoning
　　(d)　Producing cancer
　　(e)　An abnormally small mouth
　　(f)　Absence of hair
　　(g)　Abnormal absorption

Some diseases are named by attaching suffixes to roots. The most important suffixes are:

-itis　which usually indicates an inflammatory condition (e.g. arthritis)

-asis
-esis
-iasis
-osis

These suffixes all mean *a state of*, and are used in one of three ways.
(1)　They may indicate a non-inflammatory disease (e.g. arthrosis).
(2)　They may indicate an abnormal condition which is a sign or symptom of a disease (e.g. stenosis).
(3)　They may indicate a disease caused by the presence of a substance (e.g. asbestosis).

TEST

69. (a) What is the difference between arthritis and arthrosis?

(b) Diverticula are abnormal protrusions of the lining membrane through the muscular wall of the intestine. What is
  (i) diverticulosis
  (ii) diverticolitis?

70. Deduce the meaning of the following terms.

(a) Bronchitis

(b) Appendicitis

(c) Silicosis

(d) Amylosis

(e) Hepatosis

(f) Cholecystolithiasis.

ANSWERS TO TEST

69. (a) Both arthritis and arthrosis are diseases of joints. Although the terms are often incorrectly used, arthritis strictly refers to diseases in which there is inflammation of joints; arthrosis refers to diseases in which there is no inflammation.

   (b) (i) Diverticulosis is a condition in which diverticula exist.

   (ii) Diverticulitis is a condition in which diverticula become inflamed.

70. (a) Inflammation of the bronchi

   (b) Inflammation of the appendix

   (c) A disease (of the lungs) due to the presence of silica (in the lungs)

   (d) A condition in which starch accumulates in various body tissues

   (e) Any disease of the liver

   (f) The presence of stones in the gall bladder.

Other suffixes used in the naming of diseases and symptoms are:

-agra   meaning *catching* or *seizure*

-alg(ia)
-odyn(ia) } meaning *pain* or *distress*

-oma   meaning *swelling* or *tumour*

               (There are some words ending in -oma in which this suffix does not indicate a tumour, e.g. glaucoma)

-cele   meaning *a fluid-filled swelling*

-path(y)   meaning *sickness* or *disease*

-phob(ia)   meaning *fear*

-plegia
-plexy } meaning *strike* (or *paralyse*).

-rrhoea   meaning *flow*

-rrhag(ia)   meaning *break* or *burst.*

TEST

71. (a) What does an analgesic drug do?

(b) What is the difference between adenoma and adenopathy?

(c) How does a hydrocele differ from a pneumatocele?

(d) Hemiplegia is paralysis of one side of the body. What do you think quadriplegia is?

72. Deduce the meaning of the following terms:

(a) Menorrhoea

(b) Menorrhagia

(c) Amenorrhoea

(d) Dysmenorrhoea.

73. Which of the definitions on the right apply to the terms listed on the left?

(a)	Haemorrhage	(i)	A pain which extends along the course of nerves
(b)	Carcinoma		
(c)	Podagra	(ii)	A functional disturbance of peripheral nerves
(d)	Neuralgia	(iii)	A malignant tumour
(e)	Neuritis	(iv)	Bleeding
(f)	Neuropathy	(v)	Fear of water
(g)	Hydrophobia	(vi)	Inflammation of a nerve
		(vii)	Gouty pain in the foot.

100

ANSWERS TO TEST

71.
- (a) It relieves pain.
- (b) Adenoma is a tumour of, or like, a gland. Adenopathy is any disease of glands.
- (c) A hydrocele is a swelling that contains watery fluid. A pneumatocele contains air.
- (d) Quadriplegia is paralysis of all four limbs.

72.
- (a) Menorrhoea means *monthly flow* and refers to the cyclic uterine bleeding of menstruation.
- (b) Menorrhagia is excessive uterine bleeding.
- (c) Amenorrhoea is the absence of menstruation.
- (d) Dysmenorrhoea is painful menstruation.

73.
- (a) (iv)
- (b) (iii)
- (c) (vii)
- (d) (i)
- (e) (vi)
- (f) (ii)
- (g) (v)

Part six - Surgical procedures

The terms used for surgical procedures are usually constructed by adding a suffix defining the procedure to the root word for the part of the body on which the procedure is carried out.

For example:

Root	Meaning	Suffix	Meaning	Procedure	Meaning
Col-	*colon*	**-ectomy**	*cut out*	**colectomy**	Surgical removal of the colon
Colo-	*colon*	**-centesis**	*puncture*	**colocentesis**	Surgical perforation of the colon
Colono-	*colon*	**-scopy**	*look at*	**colonoscopy**	Clinical examination of the colon
Colo-	*colon*	**-pexy**	*fix*	**colopexy**	Surgical fixation of the colon to the abdominal wall
Colo-	*colon*	**-rrhaphy**	*suture*	**colorrhaphy**	Suture of the colon
Colo-	*colon*	**-stomy**	provide with an *opening* or *mouth*	**colostomy**	Surgical creation of a new opening of the colon on the surface of the body
Colo	*colon*	**-tomy**	*cut*	**colotomy**	Incision of the colon through the abdominal wall

COMMON SURGICAL PROCEDURES

CUT
-tomy

CUT OUT , REMOVE
-ectomy

MAKE A HOLE, PROVIDE A MOUTH
-stomy

FIX
-pexy

SUTURE
-rrhaphy

TEST

74. Deduce the meaning of the following terms:
  (i)   Tonsillectomy
  (ii) Gastroenterostomy
  (iii) Ileostomy
  (iv) Laparotomy
  (v)   Nephropexy
  (vi) Oesophagotomy
  (vii) Osteorrhaphy.

75. Which of the definitions on the right apply to the terms listed on the left?

  (a) Thromboendarterectomy
  (b) Glossorrhaphy
  (c) Myotomy
  (d) Osteotomy
  (e) Hysteropexy

  (i)   Cutting of a muscle
  (ii) Removal of an obstructing blood clot together with the lining of the obstructed artery
  (iii) Surgical fixation of the uterus
  (iv) Surgical cutting of a bone
  (v)   Suturing the tongue.

ANSWERS TO TEST

74.
(i)	Surgical removal of the tonsils
(ii)	Surgical creation of an artificial passage between the stomach and the intestines
(iii)	Surgical creation of an opening into the ileum
(iv)	Surgical incision through the flank (or abdomen)
(v)	Surgical fixation of a kidney
(vi)	Surgical incision of the oesophagus
(vii)	The suturing of bones.

75.
(a)	(ii)
(b)	(v)
(c)	(i)
(d)	(iv)
(e)	(iii)

SOME OTHER PROCEDURES

PUNCTURE

-centesis

MOULD, SHAPE

-plasty

BIND

-desis

INFUSE, INJECT

-clysis

LOOK AT, OBSERVE (WITH INSTRUMENT)

-scopy (with -scope)

DISSOLVE, BREAK DOWN

-lyo-, -lyt-

TEST

76. (a) What is an ophthalmoscope for?

(b) What effect would you expect the operation of arthrodesis to have on an arthritic joint?

(c) Why might an aspiring film star want a rhinoplasty?

77. Which of the definitions on the right apply to the terms listed on the left?

(a) Thoracocentesis   (i)   Surgical formation of a movable joint

(b) Arthroplasty   (ii)   Inspection of any cavity of the body

(c) Clyster   (iii)   Surgical puncture of the chest wall

(d) Endoscopy   (iv)   An enema

78. Deduce the meanings of the following terms.

(a) Autolysis

(b) Analysis

(c) Photolysis

(d) Haemolysis.

ANSWERS TO TEST

76. (a) An ophthalmoscope is an intrument for inspecting the eye.

(b) The operation binds the bones of the joint together and fixes them rigidly in position.

(c) To improve his or her appearance. A rhinoplasty is moulding of the nose.

77. (a) (iii)

(b) (i)

(c) (iv)

(d) (ii)

78. (a) Spontaneous breaking down (of tissues)

(b) Separation back into component parts

(c) Breaking down by the action of light

(d) The breakdown of blood (with the liberation of haemoglobin).

Part seven - Index

Term	Page
pneum(at)-	24
pneumo(n)-	24
pnoe-	40
pod-	19
poiein	10
polio-	83
poly-	71
post-	59
posterior	63
pre-	59
prim-	71
pro-	10,59
proct-	31
prot-	71
proximal	63
pseud-	3,95
psych-	8,13
pulmo(n)-	24
py-	95
pyel-	27
quadr-	75
quinqu-	75
re-	55
ren-	27
retr-	55
rhin-	3,14
rostral	63
-rrhagia	98
-rrhaphy	102
-rrhoea	98
rubr-	83
sacchar-	87
sagittal	65
salping-	28
sanguin-	23
sarc-	35
schiz-	79
scler-	92
-scop-	39,104
semi-	75
sens-	39
serum	23
sex-	75
sin-	15
sinus	15
somat-	13
sphygm-	40
sphyx-	40
splanchn-	31
spondyl-	32
stear-	87
steat-	87
sten-	79
sterno-	32
steth-	19
stom(at)-	15
-stomy	102
sub-	47
suf-	47
sup-	47
super-	44
superficial	64
superior	63
supra-	44
sy-	51
syl-	51
sym-	51
syn-	51
tachy-	92
tact-	39
ten(ont)o-	32
ter-	75
tetr-	75
-therapy	10
thorac-	19
tome	6
-tomy	102
tox-	95
trache-	24
trachel-	14
trans-	51
transverse	65
tri-	75
trich-	35
ultra-	44
un-	75
-ur-	27
uretero-	27
urethr-	27
uter-	27
vagin-	28
vas-	23
ven-	23
ventr-	59
ventral	63
vesic-	27
xanth-	83